The International Librar

THE MEASUREMENT OF EMOTION

Founded by C. K. Ogden

The International Library of Psychology

GENERAL PSYCHOLOGY
In 38 Volumes

THE MEASUREMENT OF EMOTION

W WHATELY SMITH

Foreword by Wm. Brown

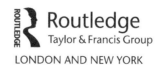

LONDON AND NEW YORK

First published in 1922 by
Kegan Paul, Trench, Trubner & Co., Ltd.
2 Park Square, Milton Park, Abingdon, Oxfordshire OX14 4RN
711 Third Avenue, New York, NY 10017

First issued in paperback 2014

Routledge is an imprint of the Taylor and Francis Group, an informa business

British Library Cataloguing in Publication Data
A CIP catalogue record for this book
is available from the British Library

The Measurement of Emotion
ISBN 978-0415-21049-2
General Psychology: 38 Volumes
ISBN 0415-21129-8
The International Library of Psychology: 204 Volumes
ISBN 0415-19132-7

ISBN 13: 978-1-138-88250-8 (pbk)
ISBN 13: 978-0-415-21049-2 (hbk)

FOREWORD

By WILLIAM BROWN, M.D., D.Sc.

Wilde Reader in Mental Philosophy in the University of Oxford

Two of the most characteristic features of modern psychology are (1) the special attention given to the facts of emotional consciousness, and (2) the persistent endeavour to obtain a quantitative statement of results. In the former respect advance has been due mainly to the adoption of the biological method. By taking the biological problem of instinct and the psychological problem of emotion in conjunction a provisional solution has been obtained of both, much as two nuts may be more easily cracked together than when taken separately. In the latter respect mental measurement has been mainly indirect in character, although the possibility of direct mental measurement is not entirely ruled out. What is measured is some physiological concomitant or other of the mental process, not the mental process itself. Nevertheless, since the mental character of the process prompts the measurement and furnishes its relevance, such measurement rightly belongs to psychology, although, of course, it also belongs to physiology.

The present work by Mr Whately Smith well illustrates these two features. In it the biological significance of emotion and of affective tone is emphasised, and by means of special methods of experimentation quantitative results are obtained which illuminate the subject in a remarkable way. The author has derived inspiration for his investigations from the work of C. G. Jung on word-association experiments. But by giving a more central position to the psycho-galvanic reaction, and introducing great improvements in the technique, he has elaborated an experimental method of investigating emotion and affective tone which is highly original and of very great value. His investigation of the relative values of the various ' complex-indicators ' is most important, and his subsidiary research on the effects of alcohol upon association reactions opens up prospects of equally valuable work with other drugs.

Mr Whately Smith has shown much ingenuity in the quantitative manipulation of his results. Particularly interesting is his use of correlation in comparing the reactions of any individual on different occasions with the reactions of different individuals to the same list of stimulus-words (Chapter V). This is likely to prove of considerable value in the investigation of multiple personality and mediumistic phenomena.

On the purely theoretical side, his distinction of positive tone and negative tone, in relation to the influence of feeling upon memory (power of recall), is a helpful one. The distinction is based upon the experimentally ascertained fact that a word which evokes well-marked affective tone may be better remembered than a less intensely toned word or may be forgotten more quickly. Its significance in relation to the general problem of repression is discussed in an interesting way.

The book represents pioneer work in a branch of psychology that has only recently proved amenable to reliable experimental and quantitative treatment. It will be helpful to the psychopathologist as well as to the psychologist.

W. B.

PREFACE

THE work described in these pages was undertaken with the main object of devising and testing a technique for the quantitative study of the emotional factors in mental activity. The actual results obtained in the course of the work (as in Chapters II, V and VI and in Appendix IV) are, I believe, not wholly devoid of intrinsic interest, but they should be regarded primarily as illustrations of the way in which the methods devised may be used for attacking specific problems. In all cases, I think, the method actually used could have been improved in some degree if the knowledge gained from the experiment had been available to start with. That this should be so is inevitable and indeed desirable in work of this kind in which the perfecting of new weapons rather than the solution of old problems is the chief *desideratum*.

The work dealt with in Appendix IV is especially noteworthy in this connexion. The curious and suggestive results there described came to light accidentally in the course of other work, and as they were entirely unforeseen no precautions were taken when making the original observations in order to ensure a definite answer to the questions they raised.

Since, for reasons given, these results may possibly have been due to the form in which the material was obtained I have thought it best to relegate the whole matter to an Appendix, although I incline strongly to the view that the existence of ' psycho-physical quanta ' which is there discussed would probably be confirmed by further experiment.

In the course of the work I have naturally had occasion to consider somewhat carefully the general character of emotional or affective states and the part they play in the determination of mental activity. I have dealt very briefly with a few aspects of these matters in Chapters I and VII, but a full discussion of the subject, to which I hope shortly to devote a more extensive study, would be outside the scope of the present work, which is intended as a contribution to technique rather than to theory.

The experiments were carried out at the Psychological Laboratory, Cambridge, and I wish to take this opportunity of thanking Dr C. S. Myers, Director of the Laboratory, and Mr F. C. Bartlett for the facilities they placed at my disposal and for the encouragement they extended to me. I am also indebted to Dr Myers for permission to republish Chapter II and Appendix II, which appeared in the

General Section of the *British Journal of Psychology*, and to Dr T. W. Mitchell, Editor of the Medical Section, for a similar permission with respect to Chapters III, IV and V.

I am also under an obligation to Dr E. Prideaux, who first demonstrated the psychogalvanic reflex to me. In particular I wish to express my gratitude to my ' subjects '—some ninety in all—without whose disinterested cooperation I could not possibly have obtained the experimental results here recorded ; I would especially thank those who underwent the tedious series of tests described in Chapter V.

CONTENTS

15

THE MEASUREMENT OF EMOTION

The Measurement of Emotion

CHAPTER I

EMOTION AND AFFECTIVE TONE

It is no part of the intended scope of this book to deal fully with the general theory of Emotion. None the less, it is desirable that I should give some brief outline of my personal views on the subject as they stand at the present time, partly in order to avoid possible misunderstandings and partly to make as clear as I can what it is that I conceive myself to have been measuring in the various experiments described.

On the other hand, it is not practicable to deal with the subject, in this first chapter, to the full limits of even the restricted extent which I contemplate, for certain of the points which I wish to emphasise are too closely bound up with experimental results to admit of convenient discussion before the experiments have been considered. I shall therefore revert to the subject again in Chapter VII.

As a preliminary, however, I wish to identify myself, approximately at least, with two of the best-known views on emotion. First, with the James-Lange theory ; second, with Professor M'Dougall's view of the relation between Emotion and Instinct.

James says, " Bodily changes follow directly the perception of the exciting fact, and our feeling of the same changes as they occur *is* the emotion." [1]

M'Dougall describes a ' primary ' emotion as " the affective aspect of the operation of any one of the principal instincts." [2]

I will deal briefly with each of these statements in turn in so far as it is relevant to the present work.

First, the James-Lange theory : With this I am at present prepared to stand four-square, for none of the criticisms hitherto brought against it seem to me to be of sufficient weight to justify its rejection. Certainly, in my opinion, no case can be made out against its main contention, namely, that the experiences, feelings or states of mind which we call ' emotions ' are caused by, and are absolutely dependent upon, bodily changes. If there were no bodily changes, if, consequently, the field of consciousness were to contain no sensations of endosomatic origin, there could be no emotion.

Nor do I see any great weight in the criticisms which have been brought against the use of the word ' is ' in the passage cited above. It has been pointed out that to say " our feeling of the [bodily] changes as they occur (*i.e.* the sumtotal of the endosomatic sensations) *is* the emotion," is to assert an identity between the emotion and the sensation, and that although there may be a causal connexion between the sensation and the state of mind we call emotion, this is not logically equivalent to identity. But, as against this, I would contend that the connexion between the endosomatic sensations and the affective component of the total mental

[1] *Principles of Psychology*, Chapter XXV.
[2] *Introduction to Social Psychology*, Fourteenth Edition, p. 47.

state (*i.e.* the 'emotion') is precisely the same as that between any other sensation and the change in consciousness produced thereby. So far as my *mind* is concerned, sensations emanating from my own body are just as external, just as much 'given *ab extra*' as those emanating from what I describe as 'objects' outside my body, and should be treated in the same way as the latter. If we say that the change in consciousness produced by an ordinary visual sensation *is* 'perception,' I do not see that we have any right to deny that the change in consciousness produced by a different kind of sensation (*i.e.* a visceral or other endosomatic sensation) *is* 'emotion.' Anyway, the point appears to be of academic rather than of practical interest, although, since this estimate of its value is unlikely to be universally shared, I am quite willing to disarm such criticism by substituting some such expression as 'is caused by' or 'is dependent on' for the word 'is.'

Nor can I agree with Professor Ward who describes the theory as "psychologically and biologically absurd," contending that "emotion is always the expression of feeling," which last "has always some objective ground." How Emotion, which is a state of consciousness or form of experience, can be said to express anything at all seems to me incomprehensible : and surely the 'feeling' which it is alleged to express is nothing but Emotion itself as James defines it and the 'objective ground' the aggregate of endosomatic sensations induced by the total situation.

Another objection which has recently been brought against the James-Lange theory, but which I cannot admit as valid, is that of Prideaux who contends [1] that the theory cannot be maintained because the emotion is experienced some time before endosomatic changes are demonstrable. He points out that there is always a latent period between the moment of application of a stimulus and the moment at which any change caused thereby can be observed. This latent period may range from a second or two in the case, for example, of the psycho-galvanic reflex up to as much as five minutes in the case of gastric secretion (Pavlov). On the other hand there is no appreciable interval between the perception of the stimulus by the subject and his subjective experience of the emotion. From this Prideaux argues that the physiological disturbance which is observed cannot be the *cause* of the emotion which precedes it. This is obviously true so far as it goes, but unless we adopt an absurdly rigid interpretation of the James-Lange theory, the latter is not in the least degree invalidated.

It seems eminently reasonable to suppose that between the application of any stimulus and the production of an experimentally observable effect, such as a change in skin-resistance, in respiration or in the rate of secretion of a gland, there must be many steps. The effect observed is the last stage in a long and complex process involving the energisation of many neurones, the initiation, in some cases, of chemical changes, the contraction, in others, of many muscle fibres. All this admittedly takes time, but it does not follow that no impulse of endosomatic origin passes up afferent paths to the cortex before the particular effect observed is demonstrable. When a stimulus is applied to a subject a wave of

[1] *British Journal of Psychology* (Medical Section), October 1921.

innervations sweeps over his whole body, so to speak. Many mechanisms are set in motion of which some take longer than others to produce visible results, but that is no reason why the general disturbance should not, at an early stage, include a reflux of innervation along affcrent paths. On these lines it seems easy to dispose of this objection, quite apart from the fact that no one has ever measured the actual latent period between the stimulus and the subjective experience of emotion.

Before passing to the comments I have to make on Dr M'Dougall's views, which I have cited above, it may be well to point out that on this theory the differences between different 'emotions' will simply be a matter of the different kinds of endosomatic sensations concerned, their different intensities and the different proportions in which they are present. That is to say, it is impossible to regard emotions as rigidly invariable entities, for these factors are clearly infinitely variable. None the less the changes induced by like conditions in like individuals will be themselves sufficiently similar to warrant description of their corresponding emotions by the same name.[1]

[1] Cf. Shand, *Foundations of Character*, p. 3. " The authors [of the James-Lange theory] rejected the common belief that the emotions have definite and persistent characters. The truth is, says Lange, that they present ' an infinity of imperceptible transitions,' and James says that 'they are regarded too much as absolutely individual things.' For if it is true that the peculiar character of their feeling is conditioned by vaso-motor and other bodily changes, and that these being variable . . . the feeling of the emotion is itself variable in different persons and in the same person at different times ; yet this conclusion only verifies the fact, clear to introspection, that the same emotion may at different times include different bodily sensations. But setting aside those cases . . . in which one emotion so blends with others as to produce an emotional state that we cannot name or identify, still, fear, anger and other emotions, though their bodily sensations undergo some change, preserve their identity."

This seems to me to lead us naturally to a consideration of Professor M'Dougall's theory, which I conceive to be one of the most valuable ever put forward in this field. He urges us to regard emotions as the affective aspects of the operation of instincts, and if we do so the whole matter seems to me to become extraordinarily clearer.

Much ink has been spilt over the question of how ' instinct ' or ' an instinct ' may best be defined. Into this, which is somewhat remote from the main business of the present work, I shall not enter. But, however much authorities may differ, it at least seems to be agreed, first, that an instinct consists in a tendency for an organism to react in a certain way to a certain situation ; second, that it is innate. Many variations and extensions of these defining statements have been proposed but are unnecessary for our present purposes. The essence of an instinct is that it is constituted by innate constructional details of the organism, such that, confronted by a particular situation, it tends to react in a particular way.

The particularity of the reaction will depend on the degree of standardisation, so to speak, of the stimulating situation on the one hand and of the structure of the organism on the other—using the term ' structure,' of course, in the widest possible sense. Identically similar organisms in identically similar situations would react in identically similar ways.

But any reaction or mode of behaviour implies certain adjustments—secretions, muscular contractions, innervations, etc.—within the organism. It is the inward reflux of the disturbance occasioned by these adjustments which produces the emotion accompanying the reaction (*i.e.*

the 'instinctive' behaviour). The particularity of this emotion is, therefore, precisely proportional to that of the reaction, dependent in turn upon the situation and the organism.

Hence it is clear that in so far as individuals are alike and in so far as the situations they encounter are similar, they will react similarly and experience similar emotions.

On one point—a point of considerable theoretical importance—I wish to reserve judgment. I am not yet clear in my mind whether emotion can be induced by the reaction itself freely executed or whether it is only the preliminary preparation, the subliminal innervations, etc., which are responsible for it. The latter are certainly efficient causes, but it may be that the free execution of certain reactions is not accompanied by emotion at all.[1] But the point is not of practical importance in the present connexion.

In any event it is clear that the endosomatic changes induced by emotion-provoking situations are amply sufficient to meet the demands of the James-Lange theory. The work of Cannon on the *Bodily Changes in Hunger, Fear, etc.*, and of Crile (*Man an Adaptive Mechanism*) and other workers on the same lines has placed this beyond the possibility of doubt, for they have demonstrated that any exciting situation elicits secretory and other changes within the organism.[2]

[1] Cf. p. 160.

[2] Compare also the views of Holt, quoted in Chapter VII and the following passage from Frink (*Morbid Fears and Compulsions*, p. 153) : " An emotion, one might say, is an undischarged action, a deed yet retained within the organism. . . . Perhaps it would be more accurate to say that emotion is *a state of preparedness* for action, which, however, in many ways is almost the action itself. The involuntary nervous system is excited in the same way as in action. . . . A state of tonus is produced in the same voluntary muscles that would be innervated to produce the action itself." See also Kempf, *The Autonomic Functions of the Personality.*

I will summarise the foregoing by stating my view of emotion as follows : *Emotion is the effect produced in consciousness by the endosomatic adjustments elicited in the organism by the stimulus applied to it, or, more generally, by the situation which it encounters. It is thus associated in the most intimate possible manner with the reaction corresponding to that situation or stimulus, and may thus be correctly described as " the affective aspect of the operation of an instinct."*

Three points remain to be dealt with before I proceed to give an account of the experiments with which this book is chiefly concerned.

First, I must give a preliminary explanation of the distinction I wish to make between ' emotion ' and ' affective tone ' — the latter being a term which I shall use constantly throughout the succeeding chapters. Secondly, I must say a few words about the psycho-galvanic reflex which has been my chief weapon of research.

As regards, then, my use of the term ' affective tone.' I could perfectly well have used the word ' emotion ' throughout and have spoken of ' positive emotion ' and ' negative emotion ' as I have spoken of ' positive ' and ' negative ' affective tone. I have abstained from doing so simply on the score of convenience. As will appear later, I have used the adjectives ' positive ' and ' negative ' to denote certain special properties of affective tone or emotion ; to refer, that is to say, to the influence which the emotion considered, or measured, exerts on the accession to consciousness of the ' presentations ' or ' ideas ' which it accompanies.

In no part of my work have I had any interest whatever in whether the emotion experienced by a subject was one of joy, shame, grief, tenderness, anger, fear, wonder, exultation, or depression, or belonged to any such category. I have throughout considered the emotion induced solely with regard to its above-mentioned properties in the matter of the accession to consciousness of the presentations which it accompanies and to its quantitative intensity.

In these circumstances I have preferred the term ' affective tone ' to the word ' emotion ' because, as a result of current usage, the latter almost inevitably suggests categorical classifications which have nothing to do with my present work. A close parallel may be found in electrical theory. The term ' electricity ' suggests a multitude of facts regarding resistance, impedance, induction, alternating and direct current, thermal effects and so forth ; and if one were writing an elementary book on statical electricity it would be more convenient to speak throughout of positive and negative *charges* so as implicitly to focus attention on a limited aspect of the subject dealt with.

I hope that, as a matter of convenience, this will appear justifiable, but if any reader prefers to substitute the word ' emotion ' throughout, I have no objection.

Secondly, as regards the psycho-galvanic reflex itself. I believe it will be clear to any reader who has the patience to finish the book that this phenomenon is by far the most delicate, reliable and quantitatively accurate method at present known for detecting and measuring emotional changes. Its precise nature is not yet altogether clear, although it seems certainly to include a polarisation effect in the skin.[1] This doubt as to its origin does not, however, in any way affect

[1] Prideaux, *loc. cit.*

its practical value, which is due to the fact that it is not in the least under direct conscious control, cannot, therefore, be inhibited and can easily be measured to almost any required degree of accuracy. It appears, moreover, to accompany *every* kind of emotional excitement, a fact which —as will appear later—is of the utmost practical value in elucidating certain problems.

At first sight it may seem surprising that this should be so, for the skin seems a rather unlikely part of the body to be stirred to activity by every situation. On the other hand it may be pointed out, first, that experiment has shown that certain reactions, such as the secretion of adrenalin, are almost invariable effects of any stimulating situation, and, second, that the free action of the skin is known to be of first-rate importance to the successful functioning of the body, especially when any exertion is involved. Now the increased secretion of adrenalin is part of the body's automatic preparation for increased activity, and, in view of the important part played by the skin in such circumstances, we need not really be surprised that some innervation of its mechanisms should be a regular part of the general mobilisation of forces or that the degree of innervation (and, therefore, the magnitude of the observed effect) should be proportional to the urgency of the demand—*i.e.* to the intensity of the stimulus.

Finally, I should like to call to mind the observations of Jung who, in the course of his writings on the Word-association Test, explains that to give a stimulus-word to a subject is equivalent to confronting him with a situation —on a small scale, so to speak. When a stimulus-word is applied, a host of associated images of one kind and another is called up in the subject's mind of a nature dependent on his past experience. These constitute a veritable ' situation in miniature,' and it is to this—in the context of the test, of course—that he reacts.

There seems, then, no *a priori* reason for doubting that the psycho-galvanic reflex will give a correct measure of the intensity of the emotion (or affective tone) elicited by a stimulus-word, or that the emotion is genuinely correlated with the latter in kind and in degree.

Thirdly, it is necessary to meet in advance one criticism which might otherwise be raised.

There can be no doubt that the skin change measured by the galvanometer is only a part of the total adjustment of the body to the situation. And it is possible that different kinds of emotion may be accompanied by different proportions of skin change ; the skin might be more affected by fear, for example, than by joy, and so on. It might be thought that if this were so the value of the reflex as a measure of emotion would be seriously impaired ; for one could never be sure whether a given deflexion represented a small degree of an emotion accompanied by a relatively large skin change or a larger degree of one accompanied by a relatively small skin change.

The answer to this is that, so far as I can ascertain by personal introspection and by the reports of my subjects, such differences do not exist in the specific character of the emotion elicited by the words of an association test. The words do not appear to arouse emotions which are recognisably different ; the subject is not in general aware of one word arousing fear, another joy, a third wonder, or a fourth grief. On the contrary, the effect, when consciously perceived at all, appears to be of a generalised and unspecific character. If it is to be given a name at all, one would call it ' startledness ' or ' embarrassment ' or, more vaguely, ' excitement,' and it seems to be identical for all words, with only very few and rare exceptions. This applies both to normal subjects and to those who were examined under the influence of alcohol.

Consequently, I believe that the reflex, when applied in this particular way is, in practice, a true measure of the intensity of emotion aroused.

In the course of the succeeding chapters, mainly devoted to experimental studies, I shall touch at intervals upon other theoretical points which naturally arise. And I shall return to the theory of affective tone in Chapter VII. But I wish to repeat with emphasis that the foregoing notes on emotional theory do not profess to do more than indicate the general nature of my views : they are in nowise offered as a complete vindication of them or of the James-Lange theory.

CHAPTER II

EXPERIMENTS ON MEMORY AND AFFECTIVE TONE

PART I

EXPERIMENTS WITH WORDS

A. *Objects of the Experiments*

THE experiments described below were undertaken with the object of investigating the influence of affective tone on the process of memory by as quantitative and unambiguous a method as possible.

It is not unusual to find in psychological textbooks statements to the effect that some such influence is exerted ; but these statements are not, as a rule, supported by anything more scientifically precise than an appeal to common experience. It is suggested that we tend to remember ' pleasant ' things and to forget ' unpleasant ' ones, and it is pointed out that we are much more apt to forget tedious and disagreeable appointments, for example, than those which promise interest and pleasure. This may be true enough, but it is equally a matter of common experience that there are many intensely distressing experiences which we find it only too difficult to forget and which insistently obtrude themselves into our memories. Common experience is, in fact, as unsatisfactory and conflicting in this connexion as in most other cases. It is also too vague to be of much scientific value.

Evidence of a much more scientific nature has been brought forward by Freud and others of his school (cf. Freud's *Psychopathology of Everyday Life*). He has found that in many cases where certain special items of experience, such as proper names, numbers, etc., which one would expect to be remembered easily, are in fact forgotten or distorted, it is possible to trace an associative connexion between them and some distressing or disagreeable experience or 'idea' of a nature calculated to provoke mental conflict —they are, in fact, associated with 'complexes.' From this he concludes that such cases of forgetfulness are special instances of the general process of 'repression.'

The reasons advanced in support of this view have, however, been criticised on various grounds ; as, for instance, that they are in no way quantitative, that no *measurement* either of 'affective value' or 'memory value' is made in respect of the forgotten material ; that the associations noted may themselves be to some considerable extent determined by the observer's interest in the subject and his views on the cause of forgetfulness ; and that the material dealt with is of a somewhat highly specialised type.

I therefore felt that it would be worth while to investigate the question by a purely objective method from which these sources of error were eliminated.

B. *Technique and Procedure*

(i) I proceeded to attempt to measure, quantitatively, the amount of affective tone excited in different subjects by certain words, and also the ease with which these words were retained in memory, thereby obtaining data amenable to mathematical treatment.

The procedure was as follows :

I applied to each of 50 subjects (36 men, 14 women) a word-association test consisting of 100 words.

The same list was used throughout except that after three subjects had been examined nine words were altered, in order slightly to increase the range of interests covered by the list. Otherwise the words used were substantially the same as those given by Dr Eder in the introduction to his translation of Jung's *Studies in Word Association*. The final list used is given in Table I (p. 32).

In addition to these, five ' practice ' words (Hand, Chain, Face, Run, Egg) were given to each subject before starting on the main list. These were intended to enable the experimenter to make sure that the subject properly understood what was required of him, and to reduce, so far as possible, the effects on the early words of the main series of any initial embarrassment or agitation which the subject might feel.

Three different methods were used for detecting and estimating the affective tone evoked by the words :

I. The Psycho-galvanic reflex. (All subjects.)

II. The Reaction-time measured in fifths of seconds. (49 subjects.)

III. Jung's Reproduction test. (22 subjects.)

TABLE I

1. Head	26. Blue	51. Frog	76. Wait
2. Green	27. Lamp	52. Try	77. Cow
3. Water	28. Carry	53. Hunger	78. Name
4. Sing	29. Bread	54. White	79. Luck
5. Dead	30. Rich	55. Child	80. Horse
6. Long	31. Tree	56. Speak	81. Table
7. Ship	32. Jump	57. Pencil	82. Work
8. Make	33. Pity	58. Sad	83. Brother
9. Woman	34. Yellow	59. Plum	84. Afraid
10. Friend	35. Street	60. Marry	85. Love
11. Cook	36. Bury	61. Home	86. Chair
12. Ask	37. Salt	62. Nasty	87. Worry
13. Cold	38. Dress	63. Glass	88. Kiss
14. Stalk	39. Habit	64. Fight	89. Motor
15. Dance	40. Pray	65. Wine	90. Clean
16. Village	41. Money	66. Big	91. Bag
17. Pond	42. Silly	67. Carrot	92. Choice
18. Sick	43. Book	68. Give	93. Bed
19. Proud	44. Despise	69. Doctor	94. State
20. Bring	45. Finger	70. Travel	95. Happy
21. Ink	46. War	71. Flower	96. Shut
22. Angry	47. Bird	72. Beat	97. Wound
23. Needle	48. Walk	73. Box	98. Evil
24. Swim	49. Paper	74. Old	99. Divorce
25. Go	50. Wicked	75. Family	100. Insult

Nothing need be said about the two last, but it may be of interest to give a few details about the first, which proved by far the most delicate and valuable test of affective tone.

The arrangement of apparatus was as follows :

A Wheatstone's bridge was used in conjunction with a D'Arsonval type of galvanometer (resistance 92 ohms) and the resistances and connexions were as shown diagrammatically in Fig. 1. The electrodes, E_1, E_2, consisted of zinc-plate discs about 2 inches in diameter, covered with wash-leather and soaked in concentrated solution of common salt. They were always applied to the dorsal and palmar surfaces of the subject's left hand, and the hand, electrodes, wool pads, etc., were strapped firmly to a wooden splint in order to ensure a firm and satisfactory contact. The galvanometer was used in conjunction with a lamp and a celluloid scale graduated in millimetres.

A 10-ohm shunt was connected across the terminals of the galvanometer and a two-volt cell applied to the bridge.

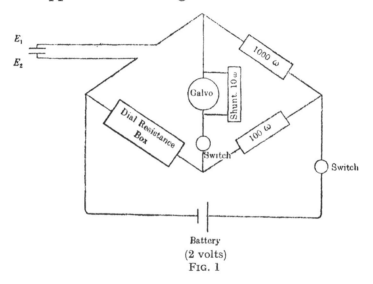

Battery
(2 volts)
Fig. 1

The general objects and nature of the experiment were briefly explained to each subject before starting operations ; he was then seated in a comfortable easy chair in such a position that he could see neither the experimenter nor the apparatus, the electrodes were applied and the patient's resistance balanced on the bridge. The necessary particulars of name, age, etc., were then taken, the five practice words given and the bridge was rebalanced. The experiment proper then began and, unless the subject's resistance increased or decreased so much that the spot of light moved off the scale altogether, the bridge was not readjusted during the experiment. (In those cases when readjustment proved necessary suitable corrections have been made in the subsequent computations.)

The data actually recorded for each reaction were :

(a) Number of the word in the list.

(b) Subject's response.

(c) Reaction-time : in $\frac{1}{5}$ seconds.

(d) Initial position of the spot of light on the scale at the beginning of its excursion.

(e) The position on the scale reached by the spot of light at the end of its excursion. (Galvanometer deflexions were read to the nearest mm.)

(f) The difference between (e) and (d). (This was inserted later.)

(g) Whether the reproduction of the association was right or wrong.

A typical line of the record would thus read :

No.	Response	R.T.	From	To	Difference	Reproduction
9	Man	8	63	75	12	(Right)

In general the stimulus-words were called out at approximately equal intervals, so far as was compatible with allowing the galvanometer to come substantially to rest between each excursion.[1]

In the comparatively rare cases in which bodily movements or other causes prevented the

[1] A complete set of data obtained from a typical subject is shown in Table XXXIII (Appendix I). The galvanometer deflexions of this subject are shown in Fig. 5, where the thick lines represent the excursions of the spot of light due to the stimulus-word and the thin lines indicate its return between reactions.

movements of the galvanometer being read with reasonable precision, no entry was made under the fourth, fifth and sixth heads shown in the above record. These effects of bodily movements were easily recognisable, for the true reaction is always preceded by a latent period, whereas bodily movements which affect the mechanical conditions of contact produce their effect immediately. A very short experience enables the experimenter to distinguish infallibly between the two kinds of deflexion.

It was found that different subjects varied considerably in the reliability of the records it was possible to obtain from them. Some gave clear, regular, well-defined deflexions ; others were much more erratic. In order to reduce, as far as possible, any accidental errors which might arise from this source, each set of observations was assigned a ' weight ' according to their estimated reliability. Observations of first-class reliability were weighted as 6, second-class as 5 and third-class as 4. Two exceptionally erratic subjects were weighted as 2 only. The weights were incorporated in the subsequent calculations in the usual way. This weighting was not applied to reaction times.

In order to make the deflexions given by different subjects as comparable as possible, I calculated the mean resistance of each subject by adding together the initial readings of the galvanometer for each reaction and dividing the sum by the number of reactions (normally 100). This gave the mean initial position of the galvanometer for each subject, from which, knowing the subject's resistance when the bridge was balanced, it was easy to ascertain —by direct calibration of the apparatus—the

35

mean resistance of the subject during the experiment.

I then multiplied the deflexions of each subject by his mean resistance (in thousands of ohms) thus obtained. This eliminates variations due to subjects possessing different intrinsic resistances. (The justification of this statement is given in Appendix II.) Deflexions were also, of course, multiplied, for purposes of computation, by the appropriate 'weight' as already indicated.

Inasmuch as the resistance of most subjects decreased during the experiment, this procedure tends slightly to penalise the earlier words of the series as compared with the later words. But this does not affect the conclusions drawn from the experiments so far as memory is concerned.

All the subjects were thoroughly normal and were drawn from the educated classes. Of the men 35 were between 19 and 30 years of age, while one was about 35 : 15 of these were junior Naval officers, the remainder were University students. Of the women 12 were between 19 and 30 and 2 between 45 and 60.

(ii) In order to measure the 'memory value' of the words, I caused the subjects to learn by heart a selection of the stimulus-words whose concomitant affective tone I had measured in the manner described above. These words were reproduced by the subjects at gradually increasing intervals and from the success of the reproductions a measure of their 'memory value' was obtained.

The procedure was as follows :

Two days after the experiment I sent to each

subject a list of thirty words arranged in five rows of six words each,[1] *e.g.* :

Long	Friend	Ask	Dance	Sick	Ink
Swim	Carry	Tree	Pity	Dress	Money
Finger	Paper	Frog	Hunger	Child	Plum
Mary	Wine	Carrot	Flower	Family	Cow
Name	Luck	Chair	Kiss	Choice	Insult

They were carefully instructed to commit these words to memory as mechanically as possible (*i.e.* not to invent any *memoria technica* for them), to destroy the list when they had learned it well enough to say it through once without a mistake, and to think as little about the words as possible when once they had been learned.

Reply postcards were then sent to each subject on the fifth, ninth, fourteenth, twenty-first and thirty-first days after the experiment with the request that the subject would write down as many of the words learned as he could then remember and would underline those over which he hesitated or which seemed to recur with difficulty. All subjects were warned not to ' rack their brains ' or to make great efforts about the reproductions but rather to write down quickly and immediately as many words as came to them in the space of two or three minutes.

In computing the results, words which were perfectly reproduced were given two marks for each reproduction, words underlined were given one mark and words not reproduced no marks.

Any word might, therefore, make a total

---

[1] Association by meaning between successive words was sometimes inevitable, but its effects tell against, rather than in favour of, my conclusions.

THE MEASUREMENT OF EMOTION

score of any integer from 0 to 10. The total score actually made was taken as the memory value of the word concerned.

C. *Results*

In case it should be suspected that the magnitude of the galvanometer deflexion is not a quantitative indication of the amount of affective tone evoked by the corresponding stimulus-word, I give here the mean deflexions, arranged in order of magnitude, which were obtained in response to the hundred stimulus-words of my list (Table I) for the whole of the fifty subjects examined.

TABLE II

Word	Defln.	Word	Defln.	Word	Defln.	Word	Defln.
1. Kiss	72·8	26. Wine	30·9	51. Street	24·9	76. Try	20·0
2. Love	59·5	27. Luck	30·8	52. Beat	24·6	77. Plum	20·0
3. Marry	58·5	28. Green	30·4	53. Carry	24·5	78. Village	19·9
4. Divorce	50·8	29. Ask	30·0	54. Wait	24·4	79. Rich	19·9
5. Name	48·7	30. Make	29·9	55. Speak	24·3	80. Salt	19·8
6. Woman	40·3	31. Pity	29·7	56. Box	23·9	81. Bird	19·6
7. Wound	38·0	32. Choice	29·7	57. Nasty	23·6	82. Bread	19·6
8. Dance	37·4	33. Dress	28·5	58. Jump	23·5	83. Old	19·3
9. Afraid	36·8	34. Wicked	28·4	59. Paper	23·2	84. Cow	19·0
10. Proud	36·7	35. Dead	27·6	60. Lamp	23·1	85. Bring	19·0
11. Habit	36·6	36. Sing	27·6	61. Cold	23·0	86. Clean	18·8
12. Money	35·6	37. Horse	27·1	62. Long	22·7	87. Ink	18·7
13. Fight	35·0	38. Evil	27·0	63. Go	22·6	88. Sheet	18·6
14. Child	35·0	39. Doctor	26·9	64. Cook	22·3	89. Table	18·5
15. State	34·8	40. Stalk	26·2	65. Yellow	22·2	90. Work	18·3
16. Despise	34·7	41. Book	26·1	66. Chair	21·7	91. Carrot	18·2
17. War	34·1	42. Travel	25·9	67. Finger	21·5	92. Bury [1]	18·0
18. Family	33·6	43. Sick	25·8	68. Sad	21·4	93. Hunger	17·9
19. Happy	33·4	44. Bag	25·8	69. Tree	21·2	94. White	17·8
20. Pray	33·1	45. Water	25·6	70. Needle	21·1	95. Glass	17·6
21. Worry	33·0	46. Home	25·4	71. Blue	20·6	96. Give	16·7
22. Insult	32·5	47. Big	25·3	72. Ship	20·5	97. Flower	16·1
23. Friend	32·2	48. Bed	25·2	73. Motor	20·4	98. Pond	15·5
24. Head	31·7	49. Silly	25·2	74. Frog	20·2	99. Pencil	15·4
25. Angry	31·5	50. Brother	25·2	75. Walk	20·1	100. Swim	14·2

[1] This word was frequently understood as 'Berry.'

The deflexions given are weighted means and may be taken to represent the reactions of a typical 'standard' subject of resistance 1000 ohms.

It will, I think, be generally admitted that the earlier words in this list are intrinsically more likely to arouse affective tone in normal persons than those which appear later.

Of the first six words, five are closely connected with sex-life and therefore likely to be of the utmost affective significance. The other —'name'—may derive some of its importance from its associations with the 'ego-complex' (some subjects reacted with their own name), but I am inclined to think that its effect is mainly due to the operation of sex-factors, for the word is obviously likely to arouse thoughts of a wife, husband, lover or other person of sexual interest to the subject.

The dominance of this group of six words is very clearly demonstrated if the deflexions are shown graphically in order of magnitude. There is a steady and almost uniform increase of the ordinate from 'swim' to 'wound' inclusive when it suddenly shoots up in a most marked manner.

The somewhat low value for 'woman' as compared with the other members of the sexual group is apparently due to the fact that it possesses a much higher emotional significance for men (mean deflexion $= 44 \cdot 6$) than for women (mean deflexion $= 33 \cdot 5$), which is what one would expect.

Satisfactory reproductions of words learned were obtained from 41 subjects (31 men, 10 women).

The words learned by these subjects were classified according to their memory value (0, 1, 2, etc., up to 10) and the weighted mean of the galvanometer deflexions was calculated for each class. The probable error of these weighted means was also computed. The results are shown in Table III.

TABLE III

Words scoring	No. of words	Weighted mean G.D.	Probable error of mean
0	326	25·62	1·03
1	23	46·26	7·93
2	77	21·73	2·13
3	12	40·00	10·31
4	22	22·89	5·25
5	12	27·35	5·48
6	31	25·44	3·63
7	38	21·61	2·48
8	93	33·47	2·51
9	102	38·10	3·64
10	457	36·93	1·34

(*Note.*—The chance that the excess of the mean G.D. for words scoring 10 over that for words scoring 0 is accidental is about ·00001. The chance that the excess of the mean G.D. for words scoring 0 over that for words scoring 2 is accidental is about ·115.[1])

These figures are not very informative as they stand, owing to their irregularity and the great differences in reliability between the different means.

Their significance can be better brought out by drawing a smooth curve of the form
$$y = ax^2 + bx + c,$$
through the points
$$x = 0, y = 25·62,$$
$$x = 1, y = 46·26,$$
$$x = 2, y = 21·73, \text{ etc.,}$$

by the usual method of Least Squares, *weighting the values of ' y ' inversely as their probable errors.* This curve is $y = ·324x^2 + 1·16x + 23·49$. For

[1] See Appendix III.

40

convenience of calculation the middle of the memory value range is taken as origin : this also applies to the equations given later.

This yields the following values for the mean G.D.'s :

TABLE IV

Words scoring	Mean G.D.
0	25·8
1	24·0
2	22·9
3	22·5
4	22·6
5	23·5
6	25·0
7	27·1
8	29·9
9	33·3
10	37·4

This result is shown graphically in Fig. 2. It is clear that the words best remembered have on the average a very much higher mean galvanometer deflexion (*i.e.* arouse on the average considerably more affective tone) than those which are soonest forgotten ; and that the latter have on the average an appreciably higher affective value than words which are moderately well remembered.[1]

If it be objected the large probable errors of some of the means are calculated to arouse suspicions as to the reliability of the curve, the answer is that elimination of the least reliable values would not alter its general indications. Moreover, the results obtained from similar treatment of reaction times and the reproduction test are concordant and, in addition, I shall show in later chapters that the results obtained in further analysis of the same material are harmonious to an extent which

[1] In the latter, a still higher affective value would have been observed but for the effects of dilution (see p. 46).

would be impossible if the general form of this curve were incorrect.

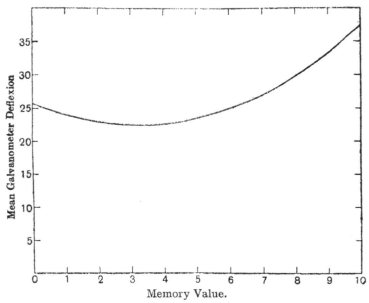

Fig. 2. Curve showing relation between Memory and Emotion as measured by the Galvanometer.

Similar treatment of the reaction times (49 subjects) gives the values shown in Table V.

TABLE V

Words scoring	Mean R.T.	Probable error	Final values for representative curve
0	11·84	·25	11·99
1	11·13	·59	11·68
2	12·13	·49	11·44
3	11·58	·92	11·25
4	13·45	1·09	11·13
5	12·18	·84	11·06
6	11·16	·52	11·05
7	10·13	·34	11·11
8	13·31	·86	11·22
9	11·39	·48	11·41
10	11·67	·24	11·63

The equation to the representative curve is

$$y = ·030x^2 - ·036x + 11·06.$$

This curve is shown in Fig. 3.

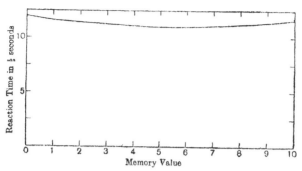

FIG. 3. Curve showing the relation between Memory and Emotion as measured by the Reaction Time.

Here again we find that the words best and worst remembered have a somewhat higher affective value than those moderately well remembered.

If we compute the percentage of failures in the reproduction test occurring among words scoring 0, 1, 2, etc. (20 subjects), and apply a similar method for obtaining a representative curve we get the figures given in Table VI.

TABLE VI

Words scoring	Failures in reproduction (per cent.)	No. of words	Final values for representative curve (per cent.)
0	35·4	82	34·5
1	30·0	10	33·5
2	31·6	38	32·5
3	0·0	10	31·5
4	45·4	11	30·6
5	66·6	3	29·7
6	36·4	22	28·9
7	20·0	15	28·0
8	34·2	44	27·2
9	10·4	48	26·4
10	27·4	234	25·7

The equation to the representative curve is
$$y = \cdot014x^2 - 88x + 29\cdot73$$

and the curve is shown in Fig. 4.

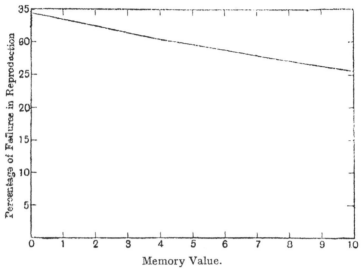

Memory Value.

FIG. 4. Curve showing the relation between Memory and Emotion as indicated by faults in the Reproduction Test.

In this case it will be noticed that the curve is practically a straight line. There is a considerably greater percentage of failures in reproduction among words easily forgotten than among those well remembered. Practically speaking, the ease with which the word is remembered is inversely proportional to the tendency towards failure in the reproduction test.

D. *Conclusions*

These results are entirely concordant with each other and clearly show two things :

First, that memory for words is influenced by affective tone ; secondly, that, so far as the affective tone detected by the psycho-galvanic reflex is concerned, its influence may be exerted

44

in two diametrically opposite directions ; the fact that a given word evokes well-marked affective tone may lead to its being better remembered than a less intensely toned word, or may lead to its being forgotten more quickly. Affective tone as shown by the galvanometer deflexion should, therefore, be regarded as of two kinds, one of which facilitates, while the other impedes, the remembering of words which it accompanies.

On the other hand, the kind of affective tone which is shown by Jung's reproduction test is uni-directional in its effects and tends to impede the remembering of the words concerned.

The results obtained from reaction times are less marked than those given by the galvanometer deflexion or by the reproduction test, and at first sight appear to conform more closely to the former than the latter. That is to say, the affective tone shown by prolongation of reaction time appears almost equally likely to facilitate or to impede memory. But, for reasons which I shall give later, I regard this appearance as misleading and consider that prolongation of reaction time is mainly an indication of the kind of affective tone which tends to impede memory.

I do not propose here to consider the relation of the two kinds of affective tone mentioned above to the varieties commonly described as ' pleasant ' and ' unpleasant.' This is a question which would take us very far and I think it wiser to adhere strictly to the necessary inferences from the experimental results.

I shall, therefore, speak of that variety of affective tone which facilitates remembering as ' positive ' tone and of the opposite variety as ' negative ' tone. To do this will imply no more than the bare fact already established that there is one kind of tone which aids the accession to consciousness of the ideas which it accompanies and another which impedes it. In very many cases, of course, pleasant and unpleasant will correspond to positive and negative respectively, but there are many exceptions to this and I feel that the former antithesis is of little value for the understanding of mental processes, because the effects of pleasantness and unpleasantness are not invariable.

The fact that the mean galvanometer deflexion for words scoring o is less than that for words scoring 10 (Table IV) is, in my opinion, due not to negatively toned words being less *intensely* toned than positively toned words and therefore giving a smaller deflexion, but to the fact that the words corresponding to this end of the curve contain a much larger proportion of ' indifferent ' words (*i.e.* words of light tone, giving a small deflexion) than those corresponding to the other end. The words possessed of strong negative tone which are immediately forgotten (and so make a low memory score) are more copiously ' diluted,' so to speak, with indifferent words, which are gradually forgotten in the course of the experiment, than are those possessed of strong positive tone which are well remembered and so make a high memory score.

The effect of this will be to decrease the mean galvanometer deflexions (computed for a mixture of negatively toned and indifferent words), at the left-hand end of the curve corresponding to easily forgotten words. If we were to eliminate these ' indifferent ' words, the curve would be far more nearly symmetrical than it actually

46

is. Accordingly, I consider that the galvanometer is approximately equally responsive to positive and negative affective tone.

Similar considerations apply to the reaction time curve. The index to affective tone is, in this case, the prolongation of the reaction time and the effect of dilution with indifferent words is to depress the left-hand end of the curve. If this dilution were eliminated the curve would slope downward from left to right more steeply than it actually does. That is to say, prolongation of reaction time is, in general, a sign of negative tone.

The curve for the reproduction test shows, even as it stands, that failure in reproduction occurs mainly in the case of words easily forgotten— *i.e.* ' negatively toned ' words—and here again this effect would be considerably increased if it were not for dilution by indifferent words.

This agrees with what is already known about the reproduction test, and the same comment applies, though less forcibly, to the preceding paragraph.

One conclusion of some importance which can be drawn from the form of the curve for the galvanometer deflexions is that positive affective tone and negative affective tone are equally definite and, so to speak, ' real ' things. That is to say, positive tone does not consist merely in the absence of negative tone ; nor does negative tone consist merely in the absence of positive tone. If either of these two latter alternatives were correct, the curve would not show a minimum value as it does ; in the first case it would slope downward throughout from left to right, in the second from right to left.

This influence of affective tone on memory is

relevant to the rate of forgetting. It is well known that the rate is much more rapid for the period immediately following the learning of the material concerned than it is for later periods. I consider that this effect is largely due to qualitative and quantitative differences in affective tone between different parts of the material.

A number of words, for example, all of which were accompanied by equal and similar affective tone, would be forgotten according to some unknown rule determined by other than affective causes—probably exponentially—whereas differences of affective tone would result in the negatively toned words being forgotten sooner and the positively toned ones later than would be indicated by the rule. This would result in the number of words forgotten per unit of time (*i.e.* the rate of forgetting) being greater in the earlier stages of the process and lower in the later stages than would be the case if affective factors were not operative. In other words, if we could discount the effect of affective tone, the curve connecting the quantity of material remembered with the time elapsed since learning it, would approximate more closely to a straight line than it actually does. It seems probable that considerable light may be thrown on the nature and relative importance of the factors involved in memory by further investigation of this point.

PART II

EXPERIMENTS WITH NONSENSE-SYLLABLES

IN view of the marked influence which was shown, in the preceding pages, to be exerted by affective tone on the remembering of ordinary words, I felt it would be interesting to attempt to ascertain experimentally whether any analogous effect could be observed in the case of nonsense-syllables.

In order to do this I used the following method : Twenty nonsense-syllables were printed on cards in block letters about 1¼ inches high and these were successively exposed to the subjects tested through a hole in a screen provided with a suitable shutter. The subject was connected to the Wheatstone's bridge and galvanometer, as already described, and was required to pronounce each syllable aloud as it was exposed. No associations were asked for and no reaction times were taken.

This pronouncing of the syllables aloud was merely to ensure their receiving adequate attention, and I found that a psycho-galvanic reflex was evoked by the process, as in the case of the word-association test.

As soon as all the syllables had been exposed to a subject he was disconnected from the galvanometer and asked to write down as many of them as he could remember. *He was not warned before the experiment began that he would be required to do this.*

D

I thus abstained from warning the subject that he would be required to reproduce the syllables without further study, because I wished to ascertain which syllables tended to stick in his mind naturally, so to speak, and feared that a conscious effort to remember the syllables as they were exposed would interfere with this.

The subject was next allowed about two minutes' rest and then asked to study, for the space of one minute, the same syllables written on small cards and laid in an irregular fashion on a table. He then immediately wrote down again as many as he could remember. This was repeated four times with intervals of about three minutes (including the time occupied by writing down the remembered syllables) between inspections. The arrangement of syllables on the table was altered after each inspection.

Twenty subjects were examined.

The average number of syllables remembered was :

First reproduction, without learning				5·1
After first inspection for 1 minute				8·7
,,	second	,,	1 ,,	10·9
,,	third	,,	1 ,,	12·1
,,	fourth	,,	1 ,,	13·8

In view of the somewhat small number of subjects examined and the unusually great differences in the absolute magnitude of their mean deflexions, I thought it better to use a method for examining the relation between the deflexions given by the syllables and the ease with which they were learned somewhat different from that used in the case of words.

I therefore expressed the mean deflexion given by the syllables reproduced on any occasion by a subject as a percentage of the mean given by all the syllables for that subject. Thus in the case of subject No. N. 13 the mean deflexion for all syllables was 7·05 mm. ; the mean deflexion of those syllables reproduced the first time (without learning) was ·50 (−7% of the mean for all syllables) ; the mean deflexion of the syllables reproduced after the first inspection of one minute was 11·5 (= 163%) ; of those reproduced after the second inspection, 10·09 (= 143%) ; after the third inspection, 8·43 (= 120%) ; after the fourth inspection, 7·18 (= 102%).[1]

The final results are the means of these percentages for all subjects. This method eliminates the danger of the results being disproportionately affected by, say, one subject who happened to give exceptionally large deflexions. The mean percentages thus obtained are :

Mean percentage for syllables reproduced at the first time of asking without learning . . .				88·8%
After the first inspection for 1 minute				108·9%
,,	second	,,	1 ,,	103·7%
,,	third	,,	1 ,,	100·0%
,,	fourth	,,	1 ,,	99·7%

These results are curious and at first sight somewhat surprising, but although I should like to see the experiment repeated on a larger scale as a check, there can be no doubt that nonsense-syllables, when present to consciousness, are accompanied by an affective tone

[1] I add here a typical set of reactions in order to show the kind of differences between syllables commonly observed.

Syllable No. . .	1	2	3	4	5	6	7	8	9	10
	11	12	13	14	15	16	17	18	19	20
Deflexion in mm. .	5	6	7	2	3	2	3	1	3	5
	7	1	3	0	2	1	0	5	7	4

which differs considerably for the different syllables. This fact need not surprise us; it merely means that nonsense-syllables, however carefully selected, are not wholly nonsensical; they are associatively connected, whether by assonance or by the mere form of the letters themselves, with ' systems of ideas ' or ' groups of presentations ' of some kind. Attention to the syllables tends to evoke these systems or groups by the ordinary process of association and their concomitant affective tone becomes operative.

There are, however, two remarkable features to be noted in these results.

First, the syllables most easily retained (*i.e.* those which were reproduced without learning and without any deliberate effort to remember them) have a deflexion appreciably *lower* than the mean (only 88·8% of it, in fact).

In the consideration of the results obtained with ordinary words I have shown reasons for supposing that there are two kinds of affective tone which are equally shown by the galvanometer and that one facilitates while the other impedes the remembering of the material concerned. If nonsense-syllables in general were no more likely to arouse the one variety of affective tone than the other, we should expect the mean deflexion of the syllables most easily remembered to be markedly *above* the mean for all the syllables, because those accompanied by relatively intense positive tone should be remembered first. The opposite is, however, the case and it therefore appears that, in general, those syllables which give large deflexions are accompanied by the variety of affective tone which impedes their being remembered—*i.e.* ' negative ' tone.

Second, we find that this effect is reversed when the subject begins deliberately to learn the syllables ; the heavily toned syllables are then most easily remembered and the lightly toned are gradually added until the mean approximates to that for the whole series of syllables.

This second effect is what one would expect on the assumption that the syllables were equally liable to be accompanied by positive or negative tone, and the results for the last four reproductions may be regarded as entirely normal.

It is therefore necessary to explain, first, why nonsense-syllables should be more liable to arouse negative than positive affective tone and, second, why this effect should be reversed as the result of deliberate learning.

The clue is probably to be found in the fact that syllables which gave large deflexions frequently seemed to *amuse* the subject. (Unfortunately the possible significance of this did not occur to me until after the experiment had been concluded and I have therefore no records on the point.)

If it be true that amusement, especially amusement of an apparently causeless nature, is always or frequently due to the stimulation of a ' complex ' and the discharge of the resultant emotion through laughter, etc., the first of these questions is easily answered.

The amusement aroused by a nonsense-syllable is as apparently causeless as anything one could imagine and a ' complex ' is essentially a system of ideas or ' constellation ' of a nature incompatible with other systems and whose presence in consciousness is productive of conflict which leads to its repression and, consequently, of ' negative ' affective tone.

The mere fact that nonsense-syllables are used, and the general situation, tend to amuse the subject and may be supposed, I think, to create some kind of a predisposition which increases the chance of individual syllables stimulating amusement-producing complexes in the unconscious. Syllables which do this will arouse a certain amount of affective tone and, in so far as this will be negative, they will stand a smaller chance of being remembered than those which do not.

The reason why the mean deflexion of the syllables remembered after the first inspection is higher than that for the whole series is fairly obvious on this view. The subject at this stage is making, for the first time, a deliberate effort to learn the syllables, and his interest in the experiment and his desire to co-operate effectively in it will invest the remembering of them with a certain temporary, but none the less positive importance. When he comes to a syllable which previously amused him he will experience to some extent the same affective state as he did when it was first presented to him. This will serve to differentiate it from the others ; he will pay special attention to it ; it will be invested with associations (*i.e.* of having previously amused him) which the others do not possess ; the fact of having forgotten it will strike him as odd and stupid and, in short, he will now be, consciously, specially anxious to remember it, instead of, unconsciously, specially anxious to forget it.

It is easy to understand how this acquired positive interest may outweigh the previous negative tone which was effective so long as there was no deliberate effort to learn.

I wish to make it clear that I do not attach any great importance to these nonsense-syllable experiments and am well aware that the results may be accidental and illusory. An attempt to throw further light on the point was recently made by Miss K. M. Banham, working at Cambridge under the direction of Dr Myers, and the results were entirely negative. Miss Banham's procedure differed, however, from mine in one or two particulars, notably in the fact that the subjects, instead of being asked to look at the syllables, lying haphazard on a table, were required to repeat them in time with the beat of a metronome. This appears to me to give less freedom as regards retention than my method and may have something to do with the negative results to which somewhat unfavourable experimental conditions may also have contributed. In any event, I do not wish to stress this nonsense-syllable experiment in the least, but it seems just worth reporting for the sake of completeness.

Summary

(i) The object of the experiments was to determine the nature of the influence exerted in memory by affective tone by exact quantitative methods.

(ii) The affective tone was measured by (a) reaction time in word-association tests ; (b) the psycho-galvanic reflex. The Jung reproduction test was also used.

(iii) The memory value was measured by successive repetitions of a learned selection of stimulus-words.

(iv) The reflex results showed a bi-directional influence of affective tone on memory.

(v) There are therefore two kinds of affective tone of opposite properties as regards memory. These are named ' positive ' and ' negative ' tone.

(vi) The reproduction test was uni-directional and indicated ' negative ' tone.

(vii) The reaction time was mainly, but not wholly, an indication of ' negative ' tone.

(viii) Similar experiments with nonsense-syllables gave somewhat analogous results.

CHAPTER III

SOME PROPERTIES OF COMPLEX-INDICATORS

I PROPOSE in this chapter to describe an investigation undertaken with the object of ascertaining, with more precision than has yet been done, the properties and significance of certain complex-indicators and combinations thereof. The word-association test has already proved of great value in enabling us to work out the differences between various mental conditions, and there is no reason to suppose that the limit of its usefulness has yet been reached. I believe, on the contrary, that it is capable of considerable further development, and that the use of the psycho-galvanic reflex in conjunction with it is especially calculated to increase its power as a method of research and also, very probably, of diagnosis.

The material obtained from a word-association test consists, first, of the reaction words themselves whose form may throw light on the psychological type to which the subject belongs, and second, of observations on the ' complex-indicators ' evoked by the various words. These two divisions overlap to some extent ; on the one hand some forms of reaction word are themselves often complex-indicators—repetition of stimulus - words, ' stereotypes,' etc.—while, on the other, certain properties of the complex-indicators may be relevant to the question of psychological type, e.g. the ratio of the arith-

THE MEASUREMENT OF EMOTION

metic mean to the probable mean of the reaction time.

Each of these groups of data is amenable to mathematical treatment, and it is just this possibility of applying a purely objective and quantitative process of analysis to the content of the individual mind that makes the method so uniquely valuable.

The precision and reliability of the results which it yields must necessarily depend on the accuracy with which we interpret the indications which it affords ; it follows that the more thoroughly we understand the properties of complex-indicators and the relations between them, the more satisfactorily shall we be able to analyse any mental condition to which we apply the method.

Many complex-indicators have been noted ; the more important are : prolongation of reaction time, disturbance of reproduction in the 'reproduction test,' too-large psycho-galvanic reflex, reaction with two or more words when the subject usually reacts with one word, repetition of the stimulus-word, misunderstanding of the stimulus-word, faults, slips of speech, translation into a foreign language, reaction with an otherwise unusual foreign word, interpolation of 'Yes' or some other exclamation before or after the reaction, unusual content of the reaction, perseveration in essence and in form.[1]

I am here concerned only with the first three of these, viz. :

    (i) Reaction Time.
    (ii) The Galvanometer Deflexion of the psycho-galvanic reflex.
    (iii) Disturbances in the reproduction test.

[1] Jung, *Studies in Word Association*, p. 405.

58

Note.—All reaction times were measured, and are given, in fifths of seconds.

Of these the first has received by far the greatest attention. The only work with which I am acquainted on the use of the psycho-galvanic reflex as a complex-indicator is that of Binswanger[1]; and some experiments on the ' B. C. A.' case by Prince and Petersen.[2] Even the reproduction test has not gained the recognition it deserves. I shall give below reasons for believing it to be one of the most reliable of complex-indicators.

In the preceding chapter I showed that the remembering of a list of words is markedly influenced by the affective tone of the words and, further, that the affective tone may tend either to promote or to impede memory and must therefore be of two opposite kinds, which I have termed ' positive ' and ' negative ' respectively. I now propose to assume this as established and to use the ' memory value ' of the stimulus-word of a reaction as a guide to the affective quality of that reaction.

At this point I must guard against the possible criticism that I am arguing in a circle, as who should premise A in order to deduce B and then premise B in order to deduce A. Such a criticism would be unjustified. My only assumption with regard to my work on memory was that the complex-indicators concerned did, in general, indicate affective tone—an assumption which, I imagine, no one would wish to dispute. I then showed experimentally that memory is influenced by affective tone and that two varieties of the latter must be postulated in

[1] Jung, *Studies in Word Association*, pp. 446-530.
[2] *Journal of Abnormal Psychology*, 1908.

order to account for the effects observed : these conclusions, again, are entirely in harmony with general psychological knowledge. I also found that somewhat different, albeit congruent, results were obtained according to the complex-indicator used to detect and measure the tone.

I now assume :

(i) That complex-indicators show affective tone.
(ii) That memory is influenced by the latter.
(iii) That there are two opposite varieties of tone.

Of these (i) was the initial assumption while (ii) and (iii) are not only acceptable on general grounds but also necessary deductions from my experimental results.

I now propose to investigate the differences between complex-indicators, not to prove their common quality of indicating affective tone.

First of all I wish to repeat that positive affective tone is as ' real ' a thing as negative tone. So far as I am aware this is a matter which has been wholly overlooked by all who have worked with the association test. The reason is obvious enough ; this branch of psychological research has always been closely connected with psychopathology, and those who have studied it have approached it from an essentially pathological standpoint. Now, in psychopathology the negatively toned,[1] conflict-producing complex is all important ; this, the true ' complex,' is the *fons et origo mali* in pathological conditions and it is this, therefore, which the psychopathologist is anxious to

---

[1] *N.B.*—' Negative ' tone is, by definition, the kind of tone which tends to drive ideas from consciousness, *i.e.* to lead to their ' repression.'

identify and eradicate.[1] Positively toned constellations do not interest him and he has not considered the possibility of detecting them. Their existence ought not, however, to be ignored by the psychologist who is concerned with the general theory of mental activity. In studying the changes in mental content corresponding to different conditions it would clearly be unwise to ignore any opportunity of identifying as many elements, or kinds of elements, as possible, and if it can be shown that positively toned constellations and not ' complexes ' only can be detected by suitable means, this fact is likely to be of value.

In Chapter II, I showed that the psychogalvanic reflex shows positive affective tone as well as negative, and that disturbances in the reproduction test were predominantly indicative of negative tone ; prolongation of reaction time I surmised to be a less definite indicator than either of the others—but to be, on the whole, more indicative of negative than of positive tone.

These opinions were based on the general form of the curves connecting memory with intensity of affective tone as measured by the indicators concerned ; I have since succeeded

[1] It is rash, perhaps, to suggest the addition of yet another term to the already so difficult vocabulary of psychology, but I think that the word ' Eridogenic,' meaning 'conflict-producing,' might sometimes be useful in this connexion. Some authorities use the word ' complex ' in a purely pathological sense, others as synonymous with ' constellation ' and to denote *any* relatively stable group of ideas. (Cf. Bernard Hart, *The Psychology of Insanity*.) The trend of general usage seems to be in the direction of the former practice and this will doubtless become universal in due course. Meanwhile the qualifying adjective ' eridogenic,' which perfectly suggests the essential features of the repressed complex, might advantageously be used in cases of doubt.

in bringing out the points in question more clearly by another method.

The material used is that gathered in the course of the experiments on memory. Of the 50 subjects then examined 22 performed the reproduction test ; of these I exclude one whose reaction times were not recorded and three who failed to complete the memory part of the experiment. We are thus left with 18 subjects with regard to whom observations were made on all three complex-indicators and who also completed the memory test.

Any reaction given by one of these subjects might be accompanied by any one of the following eight arrangements of complex-indicators :

(i) None . . . . Call this class ' O '
(ii) A ' too-long ' reaction time only   ,,   ,,   ' T '
(iii) A   ' too-large '   galvanometer
      deflexion only . . .   ,,   ,,   ' G '
(iv) Disturbance in reproduction only   ,,   ,,   ' R '
(v) A ' too-long ' time coupled with a
    ' too-large ' deflexion . .   ,,   ,,   ' TG '
(vi) A ' too-long ' time coupled with a
    disturbance in reproduction .   ,,   ,,   ' TR '
(vii) A ' too-large ' deflexion coupled
    with a disturbance in reproduc-
    tion . . . .   ,,   ,,   ' GR '
(viii) All three of these . . .   ,,   ,,   ' TGR '

(*Note.*—By ' too-long ' time or ' too-large ' deflexion I mean a time or deflexion larger than the Probable Mean, which is that value of the variate above and below which variates are equally numerous ; it is also known as the ' median.' Under the heading of ' disturbance in reproduction ' I include (i) complete failure to remember the original reaction word ; (ii) substitution of a different word ; and (iii) prolonged hesitation in giving the reproduction.)

I next divided the 518 words learned by the 18 subjects into these eight classes and calculated the mean memory value [1] for each class. The results are given in Table VII.

TABLE VII

Indicator class	No. of words in class	Mean Memory value	Rank	Classes in order of Memory value	Mean Memory value
O	138	6·7	3	G	7·4
T	60	6·7	3	TG	7·2
G	83	7·4	1	O	6·7
R	38	5·7	8	T	6·7
TG	89	7·2	2	GR	6·6
TR	29	6·0	6	TR	6·0
GR	36	6·6	5	TGR	6·0
TGR	45	6·0	6	R	5·7

Mean memory value for all reactions analysed : 6·70.

It must be remembered that the memory value is only a rough test of whether the affective tone evoked by a given word is positive or negative ; there is a marked tendency for negatively toned words to drop out early and consequently to show a low memory value, and conversely ; but there are innumerable fortuitous and external causes which may interfere with this and cause a word to be remembered or forgotten for reasons quite other than its intrinsic merits. In spite of this the main indications of the table are quite unmistakable and distinctly striking.

First, I would call attention to the fact that the one complex-indicator whose presence is uniformly unfavourable to memory, *i.e.* which uniformly indicates negative tone, is disturbance in the reproduction test. The four classes in

[1] The 'memory value,' as already explained, may range from 0 for words never remembered to 10 for words remembered without difficulty on each of five occasions. See pp. 38 and 39.

which this indicator figures are the last four on the list as regards memory value.

If we treat these results somewhat after the fashion of a team-race, giving one mark for presence in the class occupying the first position, two for the second, and so on, the indicator getting the most marks will be that which is most closely associated with the presence of the variety of affective tone which tends to impede memory, with negative tone to wit, and conversely. The marks thus gained are :

' Too-large ' galvanometer deflexion	15
' Too-long ' reaction time . .	18·5
Disturbance in reproduction . .	26·5

I conclude, therefore, that this last phenomenon is not only *a* complex-indicator—and even this has been questioned [1] — but *the* complex-indicator *par excellence.*[2]

The appearance of class R (disturbances in reproduction only) at the bottom of the list requires some explanation ; one would expect this position to be occupied by class TGR on the ground that the more indicators are present the more intense the affective tone is likely to be. The discrepancy may be due to the large influence on this rather small class of one subject (No. 18) whose learned words included seven characterised by disturbance of reproduction only and scored a total memory value of only 24. This may represent some abnormality on the part of this subject whom, indeed, I rather suspect on other grounds. If these reactions are eliminated from the class its mean memory value rises to 6·3 and the order then becomes :

[1] Cf. Jung, *loc. cit.*, p. 396.

[2] Using ' complex ' in its common pathological sense and not as synonymous with ' constellation.'

TABLE VIII

Rank	Indicator class	Mean Memory value
1	G	7·4
2	TG	7·2
3	O	6·7
4	T	6·7
5	GR	6·6
6	R	6·3
7	TR	6·0
8	TGR	6·0

I, personally, regard this order as more correct than the first, but this is a detail of small importance.

The next point to be noted is that class T shows precisely the same mean memory value as class O. That is to say : Prolongation of reaction time alone is not necessarily a complex-indicator ; it is only significant if accompanied by other indicators. This is not at all contrary to accepted views ; it is commonly recognised that reaction time may sometimes be prolonged on account of purely ' intellectual ' difficulties, arising from the rarity of the stimulus-word, etc., without the prolongation being due to a complex.

I suspect, however, that this matter is not quite so simple as it might appear at first sight. It will be noticed that the mean memory value of the class TG is markedly above that for class O or for all classes ; classes containing ' T ' have a memory value below this only when they also contain ' R.' The obvious conclusion is that prolongation of reaction time is a sign of negative affective tone, *i.e.* a complex-indicator, only when accompanied by disturbance in reproduction. I do not think that this conclusion is sufficiently in conformity with general experience of reaction time as a complex-indicator to pass unchallenged, even if we remember, as we should, that we are here dealing with general tendencies rather than with rigid rules. No one would suggest, of course, that every prolongation of reaction time, however small, is necessarily a complex-indicator, for it is universally recognised that only the more salient prolongations are significant. But, on the other hand, I doubt whether any psychotherapist accustomed to work with the association test would be willing to admit that all cases in which a significantly too-long time is not accompanied by a disturbance in reproduction are to be regarded as accidental lapses from a general rule. That there is a strong tendency for significant prolongations of reaction time to be accompanied by disturbances in reproduction has, it is true, been shown by Jung [1] ; but it should be conceded, in my judgment, that prolongation of reaction time alone may on occasion be a true complex-indicator, quite apart from the presence, or merely accidental absence, of disturbance in reproduction. If this be correct we should expect to find the mean memory value of class T somewhat below that for class O and it is necessary to account for the fact that it is not.

I think the explanation is that the class T really consists of three sub-classes, namely :

> (i) Genuinely ' indifferent ' words evoking no appreciable affective tone either positive or negative ; these would fall in class O were it not for the fact that their reaction time is prolonged for reasons of intellectual difficulty and the like. Their mean memory value would be 6·7.

[1] *Studies in Word Association*, pp. 396, 899.

(ii) Negatively toned words whose prolonged reaction time is significant, possibly accompanied by some of the miscellaneous complex-indicators enumerated on page 58. If these could be separated out from the remainder their mean memory value would presumably be less than 6·7.

(iii) Positively toned words, which through lack of intensity or for other reasons do not produce a too-large galvanometer deflexion, but whose reaction time is delayed for the same ' intellectual ' reasons as are operative in sub-class (i). These words will have a mean memory value greater than that of the indifferent words and will thus counteract the effect of the words in sub-class (ii).

In spite of this I am strongly of opinion that the statement at the beginning of this section is in general true, that prolongation of reaction time is not likely to be significant unless accompanied by other indicators, and that the proportion of words belonging to sub-classes (ii) and (iii) is small.

It is also probable that some positively toned words may be accompanied by too-long times for the following reasons :

(a) When a word which evokes markedly agreeable associations, which will as a rule be positively toned, is called out to a subject it seems very possible that his reaction time may be prolonged simply on account of the number of equally acceptable images which crowd in upon him ; he suffers, in fact, from an *embarras des richesses*.

(b) In such circumstances there will also be a tendency for his attention to be diverted from the experiment and to dwell on the pleasing ideas conjured up ; this momentary inattention may prolong the reaction time.

(c) The subject may not wish to reply with the first word which occurs to him although it may be intensely positive to him and in no way connected with a complex. For example : the stimulus-word

' woman ' would be very likely to evoke the image of the subject's *fiancée*, an image which we may suppose to be accompanied by strong and definitely positive affective tone. The first word to occur to him would naturally be her name ; but he might not care to give this as a reaction word in the presence of the experimenter. This would delay the reaction time in spite of the positive tone accompanying the word, but it would be ridiculous to suggest that such a prolongation of the time should be considered as a complex-indicator.

This agrees with the form of the curve which I obtained in the course of my memory experiments connecting reaction time with memory value. I found that the mean reaction time for the words least well remembered was greater than that for words better remembered and that there was a slight tendency for the time to be prolonged in the case of the best-remembered (*i.e.* most positively toned) words.

In view of the foregoing considerations we may regard the position of class T as quite natural.

Perhaps the most important feature of these results is the position of class G at the head of the list. It is closely followed by class TG, and the fact that each of these classes has a mean memory value handsomely in excess of that for class O (no complex-indicators) proves that they consist mainly of positively toned words. This amply confirms my view that the psychogalvanic reflex detects and measures positive affective tone as well as negative, and shows further that it does so in circumstances—those prevailing with regard to words in class G, to wit—in which other indicators do not.

Class G, in fact, consists mainly of words of comparatively intense positive tone, unaccompanied by prolongation of time or disturbance in reproduction ; if the galvanometer had not been used there would have been nothing to distinguish them from indifferent words in class O. In these circumstances O and G, T and TG, R and GR, TR and TGR would have been combined and the results would have been :

TABLE IX

Class	Composition	No. in Class	Mean Memory value
O	O + G	221	7·0
T	T + TG	149	7·0
R	R + GR	74	6·2
TR	TR + TGR	74	6·0

Here again the dominance of disturbances in reproduction as indicators of negative tone is very noticeable, as also is the non-significance of too-long times unaccompanied by other signs.

The superior resolving-power, so to speak, which is gained by the method when the galvanometer is used is obvious if we compare these last results with those given in Table I.

The high memory value of class TG is readily accounted for by, and constitutes a powerful vindication of the suggestions put forward on pages 66 and 67 above. The class consists of words accompanied by strong positive tone whose reaction time is prolonged for one of the reasons there enumerated.

It seems reasonable to suppose that the influence of positively toned words on the reaction time will be approximately proportional to the intensity of their tone ; or, at any rate, that prolongation of the time will occur with more intensely, rather than with less intensely toned words. We should therefore expect that the mean intensity of tone in class TG would be greater than in class G and, inasmuch as this tone is positive, that the mean memory value would also be greater.

The former is the case as will be seen later. That the latter is not may, I think, be explained as follows : complex-indicators, other than those here analysed, are rare in my material, but no fewer than nine are to be found in class TG ; the mean memory value of these is 5·2 and if they are eliminated from the class the mean memory value of the remainder is 7·4, which raises it to the position of equal first with class G. (Actually, if we take the mean to another place of decimals we have—mean for class TG = 7·425, mean for class G = 7·41.)

Whether this alteration is legitimate is a matter of opinion into which subjective factors enter largely. I, personally, think that it is, and I am strengthened in this view by considerations of the relative intensity of the tone in different classes as shown by the mean magnitude of the complex-indicators.

Since the Probable Means of the reaction times and galvanometer deflexions vary considerably in different subjects it might be unwise simply to calculate the arithmetic means of the times and deviations in the different classes and to use these as measures of the intensity of affective tone ; to do so would involve a danger of the classes being dominated by a few subjects whose probable means are unusually high. I prefer to express each value as a percentage of the corresponding Probable Mean and to use the mean of these percentages as the measure of intensity. I think this plan might profitably

be adopted in all similar work which may need to be compared with results obtained by other experimenters. It is equivalent to reducing all subjects to terms of a ' standard subject ' whose Probable Mean is 100 units.
In this particular case it makes no difference which method we use. The results obtained by both are shown below :

TABLE X

Indicator Class	Mean percentage of P.M.		Arithmetic Mean	
	RT	GD	RT	GD
TG	151	269	17·4	17·5
G	—	246	—	15·5
T	130	—	13·4	—
O	—	—	—	—
GR	—	235	—	13·9
TR	132	—	13·3	—
TGR	170	242	17·5	14·0
R	—	—	—	—

This shows that class TG is more intensely toned than either of classes T or G, and class TGR than either TR or GR ; this applies both to reaction time and galvanometer deflexion ; which is just what we should expect. The discrepancy between the percentage of the Probable Mean and the Arithmetic Mean in the case of the reaction time in classes T and TR is negligible.
It is possible to apply a further check to the results. If the words learned form a reasonably representative sample of the whole of the material available there ought to be some degree of correspondence between the mean values of the reaction time and the galvanometer deflexion, in the various classes, when calculated from all the reactions, and the values yielded by

the learned words only. The correspondence will not be quantitatively exact because in the case of my first 25 subjects, of whom 15 are included in the 18 here concerned, I selected to be learned the 15 words giving the largest galvanometer deflexion and the 15 giving the smallest. This was done with the idea of giving affective tone the best possible chance of exhibiting any influence on memory which it might have, and this circumstance affects the quantitative relations between the ' sample ' and the remainder of the material in a somewhat complicated way.

The comparatively large number of data here available makes it unnecessary to use the percentage method. The values of the arithmetic means for the whole material are :

TABLE XI

Indicator Class	No. in class	A.M. of R.T.	A.M. of G.D.	Proportions
TG	239	15·6	14·5 ⎫	Positively toned
G	307	—	12·4 ⎭	31·4%
T	255	14·6	— ⎫	Neutral 42·2%
O	480	—	— ⎭	
GR	105	—	11·2 ⎫	Negatively toned
TR	119	13·9	— ⎪	
TGR	107	16·8	11·7 ⎬	26·4%
R	129	—	— ⎭	

The correspondence between these values and those given in the preceding table is obviously very close.

I have entered into these details because I want to show how very concordant the results are and how those obtained by one method of treating the data harmonise with those obtained by another.

When we remember how rough a test of the quality of affective tone the ' memory value ' of a word must necessarily be in practice, and how many accidental causes may distort and obscure its indications, it will be admitted, I believe, that this concordance is remarkable and justifies us in regarding the results as possessed of a high degree of reliability.

A few miscellaneous observations concerning complex-indicators may be noted here.

In the 1741 reactions given by the 18 subjects dealt with above there are 460 disturbances in reproduction ; this is equal to 26·9% as compared with Jung's " 33% not reproduced." [1] It is not clear whether this last figure includes associations reproduced with great hesitation; presumably it does. I attribute the difference between these two values to the fact that among the 28 subjects dealt with by Jung there were 25 nervous and mental patients of different kinds, whereas all my subjects were normal.

Jung found that " on the average, 62·2% of the absent reproductions lie, as regards the reaction times, above the probable mean " ; I find only 49·2%. This difference is probably due to the same cause. Abnormal subjects will, in general, possess more numerous and stronger complexes than my normal subjects, and the more intense tone aroused by the complex-striking stimulus-words—indicated in both cases by the disturbance of reproduction— will tend to prolong the reaction time more frequently in the case of the abnormal subjects.

In view of the evidence I have brought forward above, which shows that disturbance in reproduction is more intimately associated with negative affective tone than are either of the other two complex-indicators discussed, I do

[1] *Studies in Word Association*, p. 401.

not think it is necessary to reproduce from my data the figures analogous to those which Jung gives in favour of regarding this phenomenon as significant. It may be pointed out, however, that even among his so largely abnormal subjects, it is probable that a certain number of reaction times were prolonged on account of positive affective tone aroused by the stimulus-word, or on account of intellectual difficulties. If Jung had been able to distinguish between such prolongations and those due to negative tone his figures would, presumably, have borne out his contention even more strongly than they did.

There can be no doubt whatever that for quantitative work the galvanometer deflexion is a far more valuable indicator than the reaction time. It is not under voluntary control and is not affected to any appreciable extent by non-significant intellectual factors such as sometimes prolong reaction time. Moreover, the absolute magnitude of the deflexions can, in general, be magnified to any extent desired and read with a corresponding degree of precision.

Still more important is the fact that the magnitude of the galvanometer deflexion appears to be approximately proportional to the intensity of the corresponding affective tone, however great the deflexion. This is not the case with the reaction time. It is obvious on *a priori* grounds that there must be a point at which prolongation of reaction time ceases to be proportionally significant. No one would suggest, for example, that a time of one minute, say, in a series whose Probable Mean is two seconds, is likely to be the result of an affective state 15 times as intense as that responsible for a time of four seconds. But such considerations cannot be extended to the galvanometer deflexions. Table XII shows the 100 words of my list arranged in the order of magnitude of their mean reaction times, calculated for the whole of the 50 subjects examined ; Table XIII shows the words similarly arranged on a basis of their mean galvanometer deflexions.

There can be no doubt that the order of words given by the galvanometer represents their relative affective value far more accurately than that given by the reaction time.

TABLE XII

Word	Mean R.T.	Word	Mean R.T.	Word	Mean R.T.	Word	Mean R.T.
1. Name	18·2	26. Luck	13·1	51. Wound	11·8	76. Pond	10·8
2. Friend	17·4	27. Long	13·1	52. Cold	11·7	77. Tree	10·8
3. Despise	17·3	28. State	13·1	53. Salt	11·7	78. Finger	10·8
4. Make	15·9	29. Silly	12·9	54. Paper	11·7	79. Give	10·8
5. Sad	15·8	30. Stalk	12·8	55. Divorce	11·6	80. Doctor	10·8
6. Proud	15·4	31. Pray	12·8	56. Beat	11·6	81. Motor	10·8
7. Home	15·2	32. Money	12·8	57. Big	11·6	82. Clean	10·8
8. Nasty	14·9	33. War	12·8	58. Yellow	11·6	83. Rich	10·7
9. Marry	14·8	34. Try	12·8	59. Cook	11·5	84. Table	10·6
10. Habit	14·7	35. Bag	12·8	60. Go	11·5	85. Sing	10·4
11. Pity	14·5	36. Insult	12·8	61. Bury	11·5	86. White	10·4
12. Happy	14·5	37. Carry	12·6	62. Wait	11·5	87. Pencil	10·4
13. Angry	14·2	38. Ask	12·5	63. Water	11·4	88. Old	10·4
14. Bring	14·2	39. Sick	12·5	64. Hunger	11·4	89. Bird	10·3
15. Plum	14·0	40. Wine	12·5	65. Glass	11·4	90. Walk	10·3
16. Dance	13·8	41. Choice	12·5	66. Travel	11·3	91. Work	10·3
17. Worry	13·7	42. Woman	12·4	67. Flower	11·3	92. Carrot	10·2
18. Kiss	13·7	43. Speak	12·3	68. Bed	11·3	93. Chair	10·2
19. Brother	13·6	44. Fight	12·2	69. Evil	11·3	94. Ink	9·9
20. Family	13·6	45. Swim	12·1	70. Child	11·2	95. Book	9·8
21. Wicked	13·6	46. Jump	12·1	71. Frog	11·1	96. Head	9·6
22. Afraid	13·5	47. Cow	12·1	72. Ship	11·1	97. Horse	9·6
23. Dress	13·4	48. Street	12·0	73. Lamp	11·0	98. Green	9·4
24. Dead	13·4	49. Village	11·8	74. Blue	10·9	99. Needle	9·3
25. Love	13·3	50. Bread	11·8	75. Box	10·9	100. Shut	9·2

TABLE XIII

Word	De-flexion	Word	De-flexion	Word	De-flexion	Word	De-flexion
1. Kiss	72·8	26. Wine	30·9	51. Street	24·9	76. Try	20·0
2. Love	59·5	27. Luck	30·8	52. Beat	24·6	77. Plum	20·0
3. Marry	58·5	28. Green	30·4	53. Carry	24·5	78. Village	19·9
4. Divorce	50·8	29. Ask	30·0	54. Wait	24·4	79. Rich	19·9
5. Name	48·7	30. Make	29·9	55. Speak	24·3	80. Salt	19·8
6. Woman	40·3	31. Pity	29·7	56. Box	23·9	81. Bird	19·6
7. Wound	38·0	32. Choice	29·7	57. Nasty	23·6	82. Bread	19·6
8. Dance	37·4	33. Dress	28·5	58. Jump	23·5	83. Old	19·3
9. Afraid	36·8	34. Wicked	28·4	59. Paper	23·2	84. Cow	19·0
10. Proud	36·7	35. Dead	27·6	60. Lamp	23·1	85. Bring	19·0
11. Habit	36·6	36. Sing	27·6	61. Cold	23·0	86. Clean	18·8
12. Money	35·6	37. Horse	27·1	62. Long	22·7	87. Ink	18·7
13. Fight	35·0	38. Evil	27·0	63. Go	22·6	88. Shut	18·6
14. Child	35·0	39. Doctor	26·9	64. Cook	22·3	89. Table	18·5
15. State	34·8	40. Stalk	26·2	65. Yellow	22·2	90. Work	18·3
16. Despise	34·7	41. Book	26·1	66. Chair	21·7	91. Carrot	18·2
17. War	34·1	42. Travel	25·9	67. Finger	21·5	92. Bury	18·0
18. Family	33·6	43. Sick	25·8	68. Sad	21·4	93. Hunger	17·9
19. Happy	33·4	44. Bag	25·8	69. Tree	21·2	94. White	17·8
20. Pray	33·1	45. Water	25·6	70. Needle	21·1	95. Glass	17·6
21. Worry	33·0	46. Home	25·4	71. Blue	20·6	96. Give	16·7
22. Insult	32·5	47. Big	25·3	72. Ship	20·5	97. Flower	16·1
23. Friend	32·2	48. Bed	25·2	73. Motor	20·4	98. Pond	15·5
24. Head	31·7	49. Silly	25·2	74. Frog	20·2	99. Pencil	15·4
25. Angry	31·5	50. Brother	25·2	75. Walk	20·1	100. Swim	14·2

The following points may be noted :

(i) The highest value in the galvanometer series is 5·12 times as great as the lowest ; in the time series it is only 1·98 times as great. The ' resolving power ' of the galvanometer is, therefore, rather more than 2½ times that of the reaction time.

(ii) In accordance with this we find in the reaction time series seven pairs of words whose mean time is the same, seven such groups of three words each, five of four words each, and two of seven words each. In the galvanometer series there are only eight such pairs and one group of three.

The galvanometer therefore differentiates gradations of affective tone with much greater delicacy than does the reaction time.

(iii) The first six words on the galvanometer list are Kiss, Love, Marry, Divorce, Name, Woman. Of these, five are obviously closely connected with sex-life and the other, Name, is probably constellated by the same ideas. These six words stand out head and shoulders above the remainder of the series, as I pointed out in my paper on memory. (*N.B.* The effect is very noticeable if the series is represented graphically.) Their mean value is 145% of that of the seventh word and 220% of that of the Probable Mean of the series.

Compare with these the first six words of the time series, Name,[1] Friend, Despise, Make, Sad, Proud. This is not nearly so homogeneous a group ; its mean value is only 110% of the seventh word and only 141% of the Probable Mean of the series.

This marked difference must be due to some quality, common to all members of the homogeneous group, which the galvanometer picks out better than the reaction time. This can only be a common high affective value.

A further indication of the comparative untrustworthiness of the reaction time as a quantitative indicator is afforded by the fact that the coefficient of correlation between the mean galvanometer deflexion and mean reaction time for the series of words is *increased* if we reduce the excessively long times.

The coefficient of correlation for the two series as they stand is +·470. If we eliminate all reaction times more than 100% greater than the arithmetic mean time of the subject concerned, and substitute for each a value equal to the arithmetic mean plus 100%, the coefficient of correlation rises to +·488. (Example : The arithmetic mean of the reaction time for subject

[1] For the probable reason of the very long time for this word, compare page 39. The first name to occur is likely to be that of a wife, *fiancée*, lover or other person of sexual significance to the subject.

No. 8 is 10·5, his reaction time for reaction 84 is 24 ; I substitute 21, that is to say 100% more than the arithmetic mean, for this value when computing the mean time for reaction 84—stimulus-word ' Afraid '—for the purposes of the new correlation.)

This proves that ' much-too-long ' times are not significant in proportion to their length ; for these two series only correlate in so far as the magnitudes of both are due to a common cause, intensity of affective tone, to wit ; it follows that any systematic alteration to one series which increases the coefficient of correlation does so by making it conform more closely to the variations in the working of the common cause.

It would be possible on these lines to determine at what point, in general, continued prolongation of reaction time ceases to be significant ; but this would take us very far and is not a point of sufficient interest to be worth investigating.

SUMMARY

(i) Prolongation of reaction time alone is not a reliable complex-indicator. In a large number of cases (the whole of class TG mentioned above and part of class T) it is due to positive affective tone.

(ii) Disturbance in reproduction is by far the best complex-indicator—or, at least, the most reliable indication of negative tone ; I personally regard these two expressions as synonymous.

(iii) The galvanometer detects positive tone as well as negative and in many cases (the whole of class G) does so when the reaction time does not.

(iv) Intensity of affective tone, whether positive or negative, increases both reaction time and galvanometer deflexion. In general the most positively toned words are those with too-long times and too-large deflexions ; next come those with too-large deflexions only. Words with no complex-indicators, or with too-long times only, are mostly indifferent. Words with disturbance in the reproduction are almost invariably negatively toned. Words having too-long times and too-large deflexions are, on the whole, more intensely toned, whether positively or negatively, than those having too-long times or too-large deflexions only.

(v) For quantitative work the galvanometer-deflexion of the psycho-galvanic reflex is markedly superior to the reaction time.

(vi) The ' resolving ' power and consequently the scope and utility of the word-association method is greatly increased if the galvanometer is used in addition to the reaction time. The experimenter can divide his reactions into eight classes, all possessed of quantitatively and qualitatively distinct attributes, instead of into four only.

(vii) The memory test enables us to determine the more important relative properties of these classes. It is a very laborious method and somewhat crude, but the results it yields show a remarkable concordance and it is probable that the conclusions arrived at are reliable.

CHAPTER IV

THE RELATION BETWEEN COMPLEX-INDICA-TORS AND THE FORM OF THE ASSOCIATION

IN the preceding chapter I investigated the relations which exist between the affective tone aroused by a stimulus-word and the 'complex-indicators' which accompany the reaction. I did this with regard to three indicators, namely :

(i) ' Too-long ' reaction time.
(ii) ' Too-large ' psycho-galvanic reflex.
(iii) Disturbance of reproduction in Jung's reproduction test.

I showed that, if we indicate the presence of a ' too-long ' time by T, of a ' too-large ' reflex by G, of disturbance in reproduction by R, and the absence of any indicator by O, the relation between the affective tone of words and the various classes into which they can be divided according to their indicators is as follows :

Classes				
G and TG	consist in general of positively toned words.			
O and T	,,	,,	neutrally	,,	,,
R, TR, GR and TGR	,,	,,	negatively	,,	,,

The question now arises as to whether there is any relation between the affective tone of a word and the *form* of the association, *i.e.* by co-ordination, co-existence, predicate, etc.

Sundry attempts have been made by various

workers to investigate this point by determining the mean reaction time of the different classes of association, but without leading to any very uniform or satisfactory results. This is not surprising for, as I have shown, prolongation of reaction time *alone* is likely to be a very unsatisfactory and misleading guide ; it may be prolonged on account of negative tone, of comparatively intense positive tone, or of purely intellectual factors which have practically nothing to do with affective tone at all. It is necessary to discriminate between positively, neutrally and negatively toned words before we can hope to throw any helpful light on the question. I have attempted to do so in this paper.

I wholly agree with Jung's statement that " Everyone who does practical work in association has found the classification of the results the hardest and most tedious part." Many schemes have been devised ; none are wholly satisfactory. If the system used is very elaborate and refined the results are likely to be unduly influenced by subjective factors and an immense mass of material is needed in order to give a reasonably large number of data in the rarer sub-classes ; if it is too coarse we are liable to miss interesting points which a more detailed analysis might have brought to light. The additional labour entailed by the use of a very elaborate system also greatly reduces its practical value.

I therefore feel it necessary to give some account of the system which I have adopted and of the principles which have guided me in applying it.

I may observe in passing that the first and most important principle which should be remembered throughout all work of this kind is that, as far as possible, the classification should be in accordance with the workings of the *subject's* mind and not the experimenter's. A rigidly formal system based on purely logical or grammatical considerations is likely to ignore just those idiosyncrasies which we wish to study, and so to prove of little value. I shall discuss this question of the proper basis for classification in more detail at a later stage.

The system which I finally adopted, after a few preliminary trials, is based on that given by Jung.[1]

The primary division is between ' inner ' and ' outer ' associations. The criterion which I have tried to bear in mind in distinguishing between the two is perhaps best expressed by saying that in the case of ' outer ' associations the connexion between the ideas in the subject's mind has been formed for him, so to speak as a result of objective experience, whereas ' inner ' associations are a result of what I may term the ' digestion ' of experiences by the mind itself.

For example, the associations Cow—field, or Wine—bottle, are outer associations ; one is accustomed to observe cows in fields and wine in bottles. Such associations are given ready-made, so to speak, and do not demand any subjective mental work for their formation. The same applies to verbal associations such as Long— short, Black — white, which are constantly ' given ' in conjunction. On the other hand, such associations as Cow—animal, Frog—nasty, Child—nice, are to some extent dependent upon processes of analysis, synthesis, systematisation and so forth in our minds. This last idea can

[1] *Studies in Word Association*, pp. 13-38.

be clearly recognised in Jung's classification of associations by co-ordination into :

(i) Coadjunction (a) By a common supraconcept.
                 (b) By similarity.
                 (c) By inner relationship.
                 (d) By outer relationship.
(ii) Subordination.
(iii) Supraordination.
(iv) Contrast (other than habitual verbal contrasts).
(v) Co-ordination of undetermined quality.

This principle is, I think, reasonably unambiguous and on *a priori* grounds seems the kind of distinction which is likely to prove helpful.

Its application presents certain difficulties, however, when we come to the consideration of the predicate type of association. Jung classes all varieties of predicate reaction together as inner associations, but I have grave doubts as to whether this is either legitimate or profitable.

I quite agree that predicates containing an element of personal opinion should be so regarded. But it seems to me that such reactions as Wine—red, Water—wet, Tree—green, which I may term ' simple ' predicates, are just as much ' outer ' associations as Wine—bottle, Water—pond, Tree—wood. They are equally ' given ready-made ' as a part of objective experience and are equally lacking in any product of subjective mental activity. Similar considerations also apply in some measure to very many cases of ' subject relationships ' and ' object relationships,' *e.g.* Jump—horse, Swim —fish, Make—bread. There are, however, certain border-line cases, such as Speak—explicitly, which are difficult to deal with, as they clearly contain a strong personal or truly subjective element. I shall return to this point later, but for the present I conform to Jung's arrangement.

Before proceeding to describe and exemplify the system I have used, I ought to say that I have throughout treated reactions as reversible. That is to say, I have not discriminated between the stimulus and reaction words ; Tree—green, for example, has been treated just the same as Green—tree, Horse—ride as if it were Ride—horse, and so forth.

The classes into which I finally divided the words were :

A. INNER ASSOCIATIONS

I. *Co-ordination.* This class is substantially identical with that of Jung. It is the vaguest and least satisfactory of the classes and I find a tendency in myself to relegate to it associations which I cannot place with certainty in any other class. But Jung himself allows a certain elasticity [1] and I have reduced this tendency to a minimum by omitting altogether from the classification a few words about which I felt real doubt.

I do not feel it necessary to give examples of this class as my divergence from Jung is inappreciable and even so occurs almost exclusively in his last and vaguest sub-class.

II. *Predicates.* I recognise here five sub-classes which are easily distinguishable.

(a) *Simple predicates.* By this I mean reactions in which the stimulus-word is qualified by the reaction word, or *vice versa*, in a way which contains no element

---

[1] *Studies in Word Association*, p. 21.

of personal opinion or judgment of value.
Examples :

Tree	— green.	Go	— quickly.
Lamp	— electric.	Carrot	— red.
Swim	— fast.	Try	— hard.

(b) *Predicates expressive of personal opinion or judgment of value.* This class needs no further definition. Examples :

Love	— good.	Work	— dull.
Kiss	— good.	Marry	— worse.
Silly	— bad.	Chair	— useful.
Frog	— unpleasant.	Old	— beautiful.
Home	— useless.	Travel	— pleasant.

(c) *Predicates of ' subject relationship.'* In this class the two associated words refer to some activity of which one is the subject. Examples :

Frog	— jump.	Sing	— girl.
Horse	— run.	Tree	— grow.
Bird	— fly.	Go	— boy.
Carry	— horse.	Swim	— fish.
Needle	— prick.	Jump	— horse.

(d) *Predicates of ' object relationship.'* Here the two words relate to some activity of which one is the object. Examples :

Stalk	— deer.	Despise	— man.
Wine	— drink.	Love	— man.
Kiss	— me.[1]	Make	— bread.
Bring	— sheep.[1]	Book	— read.
Bury	— dead.	Carry	— weight.

(e) *Predicates defining place, time, means, etc.* Examples :

Pray	— church.	Walk	— promenade.
Sing	— King's Chapel.	Fight	— fists.
Marry	— August.	Go	— back.
Beat	— stick.	Cook	— kitchen.
Travel	— abroad.	House	— live.

[1] These are good examples of the border-line cases mentioned above.

85

III. *Causal dependence.* This class consists of associations in which one idea is causally dependent on the other or is a common consequence of it. I have extended it to include cases in which the idea expressed by one word may reasonably be regarded as a necessary antecedent to that expressed by the other. Examples :

Ask	— reply.	Give	— have.
Lamp	— light.	Afraid	— danger.
Rich	— money.	Angry	— pain.
Worry	— exams.	Marry	— child.
Clean	— wash.	Sad	— lonely.

B. OUTER ASSOCIATIONS

IV. *Co-existence.* Associations which arise from the experience of the ideas concerned in temporal or spatial juxtaposition, including cases in which one word represents a *part* of the other. Examples :

Cow	— field.	Head	— hair.
Table	— chair.	Ink	— pen.
Tree	— leaves.	Paper	— pencil.
Home	— father.	Motor	— carburettor.

Wine — bottle.

I also include here associations in which one word forms an essential part or concomitant of an activity denoted by the other. Examples :

Pencil	— write.	Try	— rugger.
Swim	— river.	Jump	— sports.

Ride — horse.

V. *Paraphrases, Synonyms, etc.* This is a slightly widened version of Jung's ' identity ' class. The characteristic feature is that the reaction word does not possess a meaning radically different from that of the stimulus-word ; substantially the same idea is represented in a slightly altered form. Examples :

Try	— endeavour.	Shut	— closed.
Beat	— strike.	Evil	— bad.
Say	— speak.	Child	— baby.
Worry	— trouble.	Village	— town.
Happy	— pleased.	Street	— road.

VI. *Verbal forms.* I have here recognised three sub-classes.

(a) *Reactions determined by experience of the words as forming part of common expressions and phrases in daily use.* Examples:

Long	— short.	Choice	— Hobson's.
White	— black.	Needle	— Cleopatra's.
Walk	— run.	Fight	— good.
Sing	— song.	Name	— number.[1]
Plum	— apple.[1]	Hunger	— thirst.
Shut	— open.	Clean	— dirty.
Rich	— poor.	Silly	— fool.
Old	— young.	Wine	— women.
Big	— small.	Insult	— injury.
	Go — come.		

(b) *Word-completion.* A word is added which, with the stimulus-word, forms a compound word. Examples :

Wine	— merchant.	Ink	— stand.
Wool	— gathering.	Motor	— car.
	Green — ever.		

(c) *Clangs, rhymes and word-completion by syllables which cannot stand alone.* Examples :

State	— estate.	Speak	— speech.
Pray	— prayer.	Fight	— fate.
Habit	— habitat.	Dress	— undress.
Friend	— friendless.	Luck	— duck.
Silly	— silliness.	Family	— families.

[1] From recent experiences in H.M. Forces.

C. Other Classes

VII. '*Indirect*' *associations.* I feel that I may be criticised for making a special class for these associations, contrary to the opinion of some authorities. None the less I believe that it is desirable to do this. By ' indirect ' associations I do not mean " that mode of reaction which is only understandable by the assumption of a middle term different from the stimulus— or reaction—word." [1] Or rather I do not mean merely this, although, in a sense, some such reactions may belong to my ' indirect ' class.

The principle by which I have been guided in assigning words to this class is this : most associations are readily comprehensible by the experimenter ; even although they may not be what he would have given himself or would have expected, he can easily see the kind of connexions which result in their formation. There are some, on the other hand, in which the reaction word seems utterly unrelated to the stimulus-word and not to be accounted for by perseveration of ideas aroused by a preceding reaction. These must result from some past experience *peculiar to the individual subject.*

It is just such associations which, on account of their intimate personal origin, are likely to be of the very first importance in practical work and it is therefore especially well worth while to ascertain whether they have any characteristic affective properties.

I, personally, have found no difficulty in assigning associations to this class and have, indeed, done so as a rule with considerably more

[1] Jung, *loc. cit.*, p. 29.

confidence than I have felt in several other instances. I give the following examples :

Frog	— emotion.	Pity	— Blackpool.
Blue	— donkey.	Kiss	— Whitstable.[1]
Frog	— crowd.	Glass	— back.
Make	— rabbit.	Proud	— have.
Sing	— red.	Carrot	— brutal.
Dead	— coat.	Marry	— die.
Long	— badge.	Habit	— send.
Brother	— must.	Ask	— lonely.
Bed	— bury.	White	— experiment.
Sing	— feel.	Wine	— preparation.

It will be seen later that the words in this class are, as a matter of fact, distinguished by marked affective properties. This class should clearly be included under the main heading of ' Inner Associations ' but, for the moment, I prefer to keep it separate.

VIII. This is not a wholly separate class. I have counted in it a number of ' freaks ' some of which were also allotted to other classes. It includes the most conspicuous examples of class VII ; cases when the reaction consists of several words instead of the usual single word ; reaction by ' stereotypes,' that is to say the same reaction word repeated many times in the course of the experiment ; reaction by interjections, etc., etc.

When I had classified the reactions into these eight classes I counted how many in each class were accompanied by no complex - indicator, how many by ' too-long ' reaction time only, how many by ' too-large ' deflexion only, how many by both, and so on. The results are shown in Table XIV.

[1] This is presumably equally eligible for class II (c), but it is very personal and I prefer to place it here.

TABLE XIV

Indicator class	I	IIa	IIb	IIc	IId	IIe	III	IV	V	VIa	VIb	VIc	VII	Total	VIII
O	70	69	11	13	42	7	10	74	19	130	10	2	4	461	2
	80	*64*	*21*	*11*	*39*	*14*	*16*	*68*	*29*	*79*	*10*	*6*	*24*		*9*
T	40	36	5	4	25	11	8	54	24	30	2	7	7	253	3
	44	*35*	*11*	*6*	*22*	*8*	*9*	*37*	*17*	*43*	*6*	*3*	*13*		*5*
G	46	35	8	11	26	9	14	55	17	59	10	3	8	301	6
	52	*42*	*14*	*7*	*25*	*9*	*10*	*45*	*19*	*52*	*7*	*4*	*16*		*6*
R	24	14	11	2	8	4	2	14	10	11	3	0	14	117	6
	19	*16*	*5*	*3*	*10*	*4*	*4*	*17*	*7*	*20*	*3*	*2*	*6*		*2*
TG	52	37	18	1	20	9	11	24	13	25	4	5	8	227	2
	39	*31*	*10*	*5*	*20*	*7*	*8*	*34*	*14*	*39*	*5*	*3*	*12*		*6*
TR	16	15	6	3	7	4	3	8	7	12	3	0	23	107	5
	19	*15*	*5*	*3*	*9*	*3*	*4*	*16*	*7*	*18*	*2*	*1*	*6*		*8*
GR	21	10	8	1	7	2	1	6	6	10	4	1	14	91	2
	16	*13*	*4*	*2*	*8*	*3*	*3*	*13*	*6*	*16*	*2*	*1*	*5*		*1*
TGR	18	13	8	4	6	4	8	11	8	8	1	4	8	101	5
	17	*14*	*5*	*2*	*9*	*3*	*3*	*15*	*6*	*17*	*2*	*1*	*5*		*2*
Totals	287	229	75	39	141	50	57	246	104	285	37	22	86	1658	33

| | | Inner associations | | | | | | Outer associations | | | | | | Total | VIII |

TABLE XV

	I	IIa	IIb	IIc	IId	IIe	III	IV	V	VIa	VIb	VIc	VII	Total	VIII
Positively toned (G and TG)	98	72	26	12	46	18	25	79	30	84	14	8	16	528	12
	91	*73*	*24*	*12*	*45*	*16*	*18*	*79*	*33*	*91*	*12*	*7*	*27*		*11*
Neutral (O and T)	110	105	16	17	67	18	18	128	43	160	12	9	11	714	5
	124	*99*	*32*	*17*	*61*	*22*	*25*	*105*	*46*	*122*	*16*	*9*	*37*		*14*
Negatively toned (R, GR, TR, TGR)	79	52	33	10	28	14	14	39	31	41	11	5	59	416	16
	71	*57*	*19*	*10*	*35*	*13*	*14*	*61*	*26*	*71*	*9*	*5*	*22*		*8*
Totals	287	229	75	39	141	50	57	246	104	285	37	22	86	1658	33

| | Inner associations | | | | | | | Outer associations | | | | | | Total | VIII |

In this table, as in those which follow, the ordinary figures show the actual observed number of reactions ; the italic figures show the number, computed to the nearest integer, which we should expect to find if chance only were at work.

This last number is obtained as follows : if we have N objects of which n_1 belong to class p_1, n_2 to class p_2, n_3 to class p_3, etc. (so that $\Sigma n = N$) and of which m_1 also belong to class q_1, m_2 to class q_2, m_3 to class q_3, etc. (so that $\Sigma m = N$), then by the ordinary theory of probability we should expect the number belonging to both class p_x and q_y to be

$$\frac{n_x \times m_y}{N}.$$

Thus 287 reactions out of 1658 fall in class I and 301 out of 1658 in class G ; we should therefore expect to find that $\dfrac{287 \times 301}{1658} = 52$, very nearly, of the members of class I were also members of class TG.

It will be noticed that although in many cases the agreement between the actual numbers and the 'probable' numbers is very close, there are others in which there is a marked difference ; these are the cases in which the connexion between affective tone and association form shows itself.

In view of the evidence which I brought forward in the preceding paper, I regard it as incontestable that the affective classes G and TG chiefly contain positively toned words, classes O and T mainly indifferent words and classes R, GR, TR and TGR mainly negatively toned words. I do not consider, however, that it is practicable to discriminate further than this at present, or to avail ourselves of the quantitative differences which I gave reason for supposing to exist between the classes which make up these three main groups.

I therefore simplify Table XIV by classifying the reactions, with regard to their affective tone, into ' positively toned,' ' neutral ' and ' negatively toned.' The result is shown in Table XV.

The behaviour of the various classes can be more clearly seen here than in the original table. I regard the indications afforded by this table as reliable ; in most cases we have a good number of reactions in a class and it must be remembered that the crudity and liability to fortuitous interference which made the memory test, used in the preceding paper, so insensitive a criterion, so to speak, of the quality of affective tone, no longer apply here. Once we have determined the qualitative properties of the different indicator classes we can say with considerable assurance that the reactions belonging to them possess those affective properties.

Class I (Co-ordination) shows a slight but distinct tendency towards toned as opposed to neutral reactions ; the actual figures (98 and 79) for both positively and negatively toned reactions are greater than those indicated by probability (91 and 71 respectively), while the actual figure for neutral reactions is well below the probable figure (110 to 124).

Class II (Predicates) is worth considering in some detail, especially in view of the comments I made about it above.

Sub-class (a), consisting of ' simple ' predicates, shows a slight tendency to favour neutral (105 'actual' to 99 'probable'), at the expense of negatively toned reactions (52 'actual' to 57 'probable').

II (*b*)—predicates implying personal opinions or judgments of value—has a marked excess of negatively toned and a marked deficiency of neutral reactions (33 'actual' to 19 'probable' and 16 'actual' to 32 'probable' respectively).

II (*c*)—subject relationship—conforms exactly to the probable values.

II (*d*)—object relationship—like II (*a*), somewhat favours the neutral reactions at the expense of the negatively toned.

II (*e*)—definition of time, place, means, etc.—is a very small class and its deviations from the probable values appear to me to be insignificant.

In fact II (*b*) shows a characteristic tendency not found in any other form of predicate reaction. It should be regarded, in my opinion, as essentially an 'inner' association, to which general type its affective properties conform, while II (*a*) is psychologically indistinguishable from the emphatically 'outer' association of co-existence. II (*c*) and (*d*) are less obviously 'outer' but in the majority of cases they conform much more nearly to this group than to 'inner' associations. On the whole I consider that they ought to be classed as 'outer.' II (*e*) I think should be retained in the 'inner' group.

To insist on such widely differing types of reaction as II (*a*) and II (*b*) being kept in the same class simply because they are both grammatical predicates is, surely, mere pedantry.

Class III (Causal dependence) is again rather small ; its tendency is to favour the positively toned reactions at the expense of the neutral.

Class IV (Co-existence) is the first of the indisputably ' outer ' types. It is a large class and shows an unmistakable tendency towards neutral reactions at the expense of the negatively toned.

Class V (Paraphrases, synonyms, etc.) shows a slight and probably negligible tendency in favour of negatively toned reactions at the expense of the other two.

Class VI (*a*) (Verbal reactions depending on common phrases, etc.) is again large and shows a very marked tendency towards neutral reactions, mainly achieved at the expense of the negatively toned.

Classes VI (*b*) and (*c*) are exiguous and their divergences from ' probable ' values are small. They should probably be included in class VI (*a*).

In Class VII (Indirect reactions) the tendency is unmistakable [1] ; there is a great preponderance of negatively toned reactions at the expense of both the positively toned and the neutral, especially the latter.

Class VIII (' Freaks ') is very small, but I think that the marked excess of negatively toned reactions (16 ' actual ' to 8 ' probable ') is almost certainly significant.

We may now simplify the classification still further and compare the whole of the inner associations with the outer.

---

[1] In this class there are 23 reactions actually observed in the ' indicator ' class TR ; the ' probable ' number is 6. The probability of this discrepancy being due to chance is about $2\cdot3 \times 10^{-7}$.

TABLE XVI

	Inner associations	Outer associations	Class VII	Totals
Positively toned	297	215	16	528
	279	*224*	*27*	
Neutral . .	351	352	11	714
	380	*298*	*37*	
Negatively toned	230	127	59	416
	219	*172*	*22*	
Totals . .	878	694	86	1658

It is clear that inner associations contain a marked preponderance of positively and negatively toned reactions and a marked lack of neutral reactions ; outer associations favour the neutral reactions chiefly at the expense of the negatively toned.

As I have already observed, I consider that class VII should be included among inner associations. I have kept it distinct up to this point, partly because its type of association is, by definition, somewhat obscure and partly because I wanted to show the tendencies of inner associations without there being any question of their being unduly influenced by the inclusion of reaction forms which might appear of dubious eligibility. When class VII is thus included the figures become :

TABLE XVII

	Inner associations	Outer associations	Totals
Positively toned	313	215	528
	306	*224*	
Neutral . .	362	352	714
	417	*298*	
Negatively toned	289	127	416
	241	*172*	
Totals . .	964	694	1658

Inner associations show the same characteristics as before, but more markedly with regard to negatively toned reaction and less so with regard to positively toned.

Finally, I shall assume that my contentions as regards predicate forms are warranted and shall transfer classes II (*a*), II (*c*) and II (*d*) to the outer associations. The figures then become :

TABLE XVIII

	Inner associations	Outer associations	Totals
Positively toned	183	345	528
	176	*354*	
Neutral . .	173	541 [1]	714
	240	*475*	
Negatively toned	199	217	416
	139	*274*	
Totals . .	555	1103	1658

This again greatly increases the relative predominance of negatively toned reactions among the inner associations ; it slightly reduces the relative differences between actual and probable figures for outer associations of all three kinds —they are, in fact, slightly diluted by the addition of a number of reactions distributed in close accordance with probability.

It may be convenient to keep these predicate classes II (*a*), II (*c*) and II (*d*) with the other predicates for certain purposes, but I think there can be no doubt that if we are considering reactions from the affective point of view, their proper place is with the outer associations. And, after all, it is the affective tone which we are

[1] The chance of this difference between the actual and probable figures being accidental is about one in two million. See Appendix III.

seeking in all practical applications of association methods ; reactions unaccompanied by it are of no great value, they do not lead to significant complexes of pathological importance or even to constellations of theoretical interest.

The affectively toned reactions are the important reactions, especially—for clinical work—those which are negatively toned. If, therefore, we are desirous of ' summing up ' a subject in the way which is sometimes attempted by study of the ' reaction-type,' it is important that we should adopt the system of classification which will most clearly show the relative number of reactions constellated by ' complexes ' — *i.e.* which are negatively toned—and that we should know which classes are likely to contain the greatest proportion of such reactions.

The best way to do this would be to use all three complex-indicators, viz. : reaction time, psycho-galvanic reflex and the reproduction test. A complete analysis into the ' indicator classes ' can then be made. But it may well be that external circumstances may not permit of the application of all, or indeed of any, of these tests. In such a case we have only the *form* of the reactions to fall back on and I think it is clear that the relative proportion of complex-determined reactions will be much more clearly shown if we adopt the system of classification which I have here advocated (viz. separation of predicate forms into ' outer ' and ' inner ' and the inclusion of all the very indirect and ' personally ' constellated reactions of my class VII —under the head of ' inner associations '), than if we adhere to the scheme used by Jung. The proportion of inner associations to outer will then afford some measure of the subject's

G

' complexity '—if I may coin a word to denote possession of complexes.

My figures show that for normal subjects the proportion of inner to outer associations is almost precisely 1 to 2 and any proportion much greater than this is likely to mean a correspondingly large number of negatively-toned, complex-determined reactions and therefore to be significant. The most important classes from this point of view are II (b) and VII. Class I is somewhat significant, although much less so, and the figures for class VIII show that ' freaks ' are very noteworthy.

I do not claim that this method is anything but very rough, only that it is likely to be less misleading than existing methods.

At the risk of prolixity and repetition I wish to emphasise the point of view indicated in the preceding paragraphs. My contention is that no system of classifying reactions can be of any value unless it is based on the nature of the psychical processes which determine those reactions rather than on the verbal or grammatical form which they may take. The different forms are only of interest in so far as they can be correlated with significant psychical conditions of one kind or another ; apart from this they are merely academic and sterile.

But we are beginning to realise with increasing clearness that affective tone is the dominant factor in all mental activity ; complexes owe their power and their very existence solely to its operation ; its distribution, so to speak, is the all-important determinant of the mental state of the individual. Consequently any sound scheme of classification must, in the last analysis, be based upon the affective tone concomitant to the reactions concerned and affective considerations must override all others of a formal and academic nature.

Before proceeding to the interpretation of these results I wish to enlarge for a moment upon the concept of ' positive ' and ' negative ' affective tone which I have introduced into these studies. I do not propose to discuss them exhaustively here but I feel that it will be wise to consolidate my position and to guard against possible criticism by recalling the terms in which I defined the words.

It is important that the distinction drawn between the two kinds of affective tone should be a valid distinction and truly relevant to mental processes as they actually occur ; also that the criterion chosen for establishing the presence of each kind of tone should be of a nature to effect such a valid discrimination.

It will be remembered that I defined negative tone as that variety which tends to repel attention, or to impede the accession to consciousness of the ideas to which it is concomitant ; positive tone was defined as the opposite to this.

I think it will be conceded that the operation of negative tone, so defined, is clearly identical, in nature though not necessarily in intensity, with the process commonly known as ' repression.' The operation of positive tone is, of course, simply the reverse of this.

I identified these two varieties of tone as concomitant to certain classes of reaction by measuring quantitatively the effects of their operation ; that is to say I actually measured the tendency for the stimulus-words of the reactions concerned to have their accession to consciousness impeded—*i.e.* to be ' forgotten.'

I submit that this purely empirical procedure yields results which are strictly relevant to mental processes as actually met with and, notably, to those varieties of them which are particularly studied by psychopathologists.

After this digression we may return to the consideration of the results recorded in Tables XIV–XVIII.

I may as well say at the outset that I have doubts as to whether the study of ' reaction types ' based upon any system of classifying reactions is likely to prove of great practical value apart from research work. But Jung and other authorities appear to consider it important and potentially valuable and it may prove to be so for certain purposes—*e.g.* diagnosis —but only in so far as we properly understand the significance of the different forms of reaction.

Inspection of Table XV shows that the reaction classes may be divided into two main groups :

> (i) Those which favour ' toned ' reactions at the expense of ' untoned.' The principal numbers of this group are classes I, II (*b*), II (*e*), III, VII and (VIII).
>
> (ii) Those which favour ' untoned ' reactions at the expense of ' toned.' The chief examples here are II (*a*), II (*d*), IV and VI (*a*).

Class V is rather indeterminate and conforms so closely to the probable figures that I shall not consider it further ; classes II (*c*), VI (*b*) and VI (*c*) are too small to afford a reliable basis for discussion.

Of the classes comprising the first group all are incontestably ' inner ' associations ; in the second group classes IV and VI (*a*) are equally undoubtedly ' outer ' associations and I have given reasons for holding that classes II (a) and II (d) should also be reckoned as ' outer.'

All this is in accordance with expectation ; outer reactions are obviously of a more superficial type than inner, the stimulus-word does not penetrate so deeply into the mind, so to speak, because a suitable reaction is easily found. This is rather a loose way of speaking ; it would perhaps be more accurate to say that the subject follows the line of least resistance and gives the reaction which combines the maximum of accessibility with the minimum of negative tone. The more accessible, the more familiar, the more superficial an idea associated with the stimulus-word is, the greater the chance of ' dodging ' negative tone. Or, better, the accessible and familiar associated words are just those which, by virtue of the association having been formed in countless varying contexts, possess no specific tone.

This is well borne out by the figures for the principal classes. The most superficial class of all is class VI (a), consisting of reactions conditioned by common phrases, antitheses, etc. Such reactions can take place with the minimum of attention to the true ' inwardness ' of the stimulus-word ; they are as nearly as possible purely automatic. The actual number of neutral reactions in this class (160) is 131% of the probable number (122), while the toned reactions only amount to 77% of the probable number.

Class IV (Co-existence) is less superficial ; the formation of such reactions requires rather more attention, although no contemplation of the attributes of the object [1] suggested by the

---

[1] *N.B.*—Stimulus-words giving rise to co-existence reactions are, of necessity, almost invariably concretes.

stimulus-word is necessary. The corresponding figures to those quoted above are : neutral reactions 122%, toned reactions 77%.

Class II (a) (Simple Predicates) again demand for their formation somewhat closer attention still to the stimulus-word, for the simple predicate is essentially an apprehended and named attribute. The figures here are 105% and 95% respectively.

Class II (d) does not conform unless it be reckoned more superficial than II (a). It is difficult to say whether this is correct, but it is obviously not a preposterous suggestion, and the figures (109% and 92%) differ but slightly from the preceding ones.

Similarly with the inner reactions we find that the tendency for tone to show itself is substantially proportional to the extent to which the reaction is personal and peculiar to the subject, or in other words to the degree of its 'innerness.'

Thus class I (Co-ordination) is comparatively superficial. The figures are : neutral reactions 89% of the probable number, toned reactions 109%.

Class III (Causal Dependence) is distinctly of a more 'inner' nature. The figures are 72% and 122%.

Class II (b) is clearly much more personal, consisting as it does of reactions containing an expression of personal opinion. The figures are 50% and 137% respectively.

Class VII is by definition the most intimately personal of all (cf. section 4 (c)) and accordingly we find that the figures are 30% and 153%.

Class II (e) is rather small and not very easy to place : in my judgment it should probably be located between I and III. The figures are 82% and 110%.

Class VIII is much too small to give reliable figures in this connexion ; inasmuch as it contains a number of reactions taken from class VII and a few ' stereotypes,' it is highly personal, but is diluted to some extent by polyverbal reactions, which, although significant, are not quite so obviously peculiar to the individual subject as are the numbers of class VII ; the corresponding figures are 36% and 147%.

Thus we find, as we progress from class VI (a), the most superficial of all, to class VII the most peculiar, the most personal, the most truly inner, a steady increase in the numbers of toned reactions and a steady decrease in the number of neutral reactions. These figures are shown in Table XIX.

TABLE XIX

Class	Description	Actual number of reactions shown as a percentage of the probable number	
		Neutral	Toned
VI (a)	Purely verbal	131%	77%
IV	Co-existence	122%	77%
II (d)	Object relationship	109%	92%
II (a)	Simple predicate	105%	95%
I	Co-ordination	89%	109%
III	Causal dependence	72%	122%
II (b)	Predicates of opinion	50%	137%
VII	Indirect, personal	30%	153%

If we confine ourselves to the consideration of *negative* tone only we have :

TABLE XX

| Class | Actual number of reactions shown as a percentage of the probable number | |
	Neutral	Negatively toned
VI (a)	131%	58%
IV	122%	64%
II (d)	109%	80%
II (a)	105%	91%
I	89%	111%
III	72%	(100%)
II (b)	50%	174%
VII	30%	268%

Class III fails to conform in this case but the general agreement with Table XIX is excellent.

I contend that this alone is sufficient justification for the system of classification which I have adopted and if it be considered with the other evidence I have adduced the soundness of this system will, I think, be unmistakably apparent.

Anyone who has done any practical surveying will know what is meant by ' closing a traverse.' I start, let us say, from point A, I take observations and calculate the position of point B, thence I work to C, from C to D, from D to E and finally back again to A. If the position of A thus computed coincides with its known position from which I started I conclude that the intermediate measurements and calculations have been correctly made ; it is an extraordinarily delicate check, as anyone who has tried it will admit.

A somewhat similar check can be applied to the investigations embodied in this chapter and the two which preceded it.

I started by showing that affective tone, as detected and measured by certain indicators, exerted an influence on the remembering of the words to which it was concomitant ; I next used this fact as a means of differentiation between different combinations of these indicators and for determining their affective properties ; finally I applied the results of this process of differentiation to the study of the relation between the various types of associations and the affective tone concomitant to them.

If these methods are valid and if the tendency I have found for negatively toned reactions to predominate among inner associations and neutral reactions among outer is a real tendency, we should expect the mean ' memory value ' of learned words belonging to the former class to be smaller than that of words belonging to the latter. This would constitute a ' check back ' on to my starting-point.

I have accordingly computed the mean memory value for inner and outer associations (classified according to the system I have been advocating) ; the values are 6·5 and 7·5 respectively.[1]

Thus we see that starting from Memory,

[1] If an analogous system of marking be employed which takes account, not of a word being well remembered or quickly forgotten, but of its being *one or the other as opposed to being moderately well remembered* (equally high marks being given for immediate forgetting as for permanent retention), figures of merit for inner as compared with outer associations can be obtained which indicate the affective ' importance ' or ' potency,' so to speak, of the reactions (as regards memory) irrespective of their ' sense ' or ' direction.' The figures of merit thus obtained are 9·1 for inner associations and 9·2 for outer associations. The difference is negligible, and the inference is that the affective forces concomitant to inner associations are, in general, uni-directional and predominantly ' *negative.*' If they were ambi-directional the figure of merit of inner associations would be substantially higher than that for outer associations. That is to say, the ' innerness ' of an association is, on the whole, an indication of negative tone.

proceeding to Complex-indicators, working from these to the Forms of Associations and finally back again to Memory, the results are uniformly concordant.

When we remember the many fortuitous causes which conspire to make the memory test insensitive and the considerable scope for error which there is in classifying the forms of associations, this ' closing of the traverse ' can, I think, fairly be claimed as remarkably satisfactory evidence of the reliability of the methods used and the validity of the conclusions obtained.

Finally, it is necessary to consider the bearing of these conclusions as to the form of association on the practical use of the association test. I have already said that I do not think it is likely to be very great, but it cannot be doubted that the more thoroughly the test is understood by those who use it and the more perfectly the relations between its various features are appreciated, the better the results obtained are likely to be. And I believe that it may well prove a very valuable weapon for purely research purposes.

The test is sometimes used as a preliminary to psycho-analysis ; the physician applies it in order to gain some idea of the general mental type of the patient and some guide to his principal complexes. He is essentially on the look out for pointers which shall tell him where he may most profitably begin the detailed exploration of the patient's mind ; he wishes to shorten his labours by selecting the most promising *point de départ* for the analysis. It may be doubted whether the method is as yet fully appreciated, but some psycho-analysts value it highly.

The success of the test and the amount of information to be gained from it must necessarily depend to a large extent on the experience of the physician. It is hardly a matter which can be reduced to a rigid formula ; the conclusions drawn must rather result from a gradual process of correlating all kinds of indications given by the test with knowledge as to their import derived from various sources. The ease and certainty with which the physician can sum up his patient must be strictly limited by the extent and accuracy of this knowledge ; it is all important that he should know, as precisely as possible, which indications are noteworthy and which are not.

So far as the form of the association goes there can be no doubt, in my opinion, that the most significant characteristic is the degree of idiosyncrasy of the reaction word. Stereotypes and multiverbal reactions (part of my class VIII) and very indirect ' personal ' associations (class VII) are the most significant of all ; then come predicate forms involving an expression of personal opinion or judgment of value. Outer associations, especially those verbal forms constellated by common phrases of everyday life, are quite insignificant, though I think it probable that the true ' clang '—as opposed to the rhyme—is often a complex-indicator.

In attempting to ascertain the general tendency for stimulus-words to elicit emotionally toned reactions the best guide, so far as the form of associations is concerned, is probably the percentage of inner associations ; the word ' inner ' being defined as I have advocated above.

THE MEASUREMENT OF EMOTION

Summary

(i) Comparison of the verbal forms of association with the accompanying complex-indicators shows that there are marked differences of affective value between the various forms.

(ii) Simple predicates should not be classed as 'inner' associations.

(iii) Indirect 'personal' associations, as here defined, are highly significant. So also are predicates giving expression of personal opinion, etc.

(iv) The system of classification here suggested yields results which harmonise very well with previous experiments and enables associations to be arranged in a graded series of affective importance.

(v) The 'innerness' of an association is, in the main, an index of negative tone.

CHAPTER V

EXPERIMENTS ON THE ASSOCIATION TEST AS A CRITERION OF INDIVIDUALITY

THE object of the next series of experiments was to ascertain whether, and to what extent, the distribution of affective tone evoked in the course of a word-association test is uniquely characteristic of the subject concerned. For reasons which I shall give later I consider this question to be of considerable importance.

In order to investigate the point, I induced six subjects to undergo repeated tests :

Subject	P1	was tested on	6	occasions.
,,	P2	,,	8	,,
,,	P3	,,	8	,,
,,	P4	,,	6	,,
,,	P5	,,	10	,,
,,	P6	,,	6	,,

The general procedure was substantially the same as that described in Chapter II, but I did not take reaction times and relied solely on the psycho-galvanic reflex as a measure of the affective tone evolved. I did this partly because I believe the reflex to be far more reliable than reaction time and partly because I wished, for external reasons, to shorten, as much as possible, both the experiments themselves and the subsequent calculations.

I also made certain changes in the list of words used. It is obvious that to use a list containing any considerable number of words likely to arouse intense affective tone in *all* subjects would tend to obscure the individual differences which I was anxious to investigate. The ideal would be to use a list containing only words of no universal interest which would, therefore, only evoke affective tone by virtue of their associations with experiences peculiar to the individual ; but this is scarcely practicable.

As an approximation to this I deleted from my original list the twenty words which, in my previous experiments, had aroused the most intense affective tone in subjects as a whole. These, in the order in which they appeared in my original list, were :

Woman, Dance, Proud, Habit, Pray, Money, Despise, War, Child, Marry, Fight, Family, Name, Afraid, Love, Kiss, State, Happy, Wound, Divorce.

I replaced these by the following twenty words which I judged less likely to arouse intensive affective tone in the average subject :

Window, Pay, Mountain, Justice, Hat, Paint, Wild, Month, Brown, Dog, Help, Apple, Waste, Fast, Purpose, Knife, House, Coal, Fire, Hotel.

The list then ran as follows :

TABLE XXI

1. Head	26. Blue	51. Frog	76. Wait
2. Green	27. Lamp	52. Try	77. Cow
3. Water	28. Carry	53. Hunger	78. Waste
4. Sing	29. Bread	54. White	79. Luck
5. Dead	30. Rich	55. Brown	80. Horse
6. Long	31. Tree	56. Speak	81. Table
7. Ship	32. Jump	57. Pencil	82. Work
8. Make	33. Pity	58. Sad	83. Brother
9. Window	34. Yellow	59. Plum	84. Fast
10. Friend	35. Street	60. Dog	85. Purpose
11. Cook	36. Bury	61. Home	86. Chair
12. Ask	37. Salt	62. Nasty	87. Worry
13. Cold	38. Dress	63. Glass	88. Knife
14. Stalk	39. Justice	64. Help	89. Motor
15. Pay	40. Hat	65. Wine	90. Clean
16. Village	41. Paint	66. Big	91. Bag
17. Pond	42. Silly	67. Carrot	92. Choice
18. Sick	43. Book	68. Give	93. Bed
19. Mountain	44. Wild	69. Doctor	94. House
20. Bring	45. Finger	70. Travel	95. Coal
21. Ink	46. Month	71. Flower	96. Shut
22. Angry	47. Bird	72. Beat	97. Fire
23. Needle	48. Walk	73. Box	98. Evil
24. Swim	49. Paper	74. Old	99. Hotel
25. Go	50. Wicked	75. Apple	100. Insult

Each time that I tested a given subject I called out the words of the list in a different order. Thus I first gave them in the order shown above, next backwards, then in the order 1, 3, 5, 7 . . . 99, 2, 4, 6, 8 . . . 100 ; for the third test I used the order 100, 98, 96 . . . 2, 99, 97, 95 . . . 1 ; and similar systematic alterations of order were made for each test.

There were several reasons for doing this. In the first place, I wished to eliminate, as far as possible, any effects due to perseveration, and reversing the order of the words is calculated to do this to some extent. Secondly, I feared that if I always used the same order the subjects would soon begin to remember which word was coming next, and that this would be apt to interfere with the success of the experiment. Thirdly, some subjects have a tendency to ' settle down ' in the course of the experiment and to give smaller reactions towards the end than at the beginning, while others behave in the opposite way.

By varying the order of the words such sources of error can be minimised.

In order to eliminate the danger of the results being unduly influenced by tests the absolute magnitude of whose reactions might happen to be abnormally large or small, I adopted the same ' percentage method ' which I used in my experiments on nonsense-syllables. That is to say, I expressed each reaction as a percentage of the arithmetic mean of the series to which it belonged ; each series, therefore, was of equal weight in determining the final results, no matter what the absolute magnitude of its mean reaction might be.

The tests on each subject were carried out at intervals of two or three days.

In order to ascertain the average consistency of individual subjects—the extent, that is to say, to which an individual's reactions on one occasion resembled his reactions on another— I divided the tests for each subject into two equal groups, taking the first three, four or five tests, as the case might be, as one group, and the last three, four or five as the other group. Thus for subject P1 the first group consisted of tests 1, 2 and 3 and the other of tests 4, 5 and 6, while for subject P5 one group consisted of tests 1, 2, 3, 4 and 5, and the other of tests 6, 7, 8, 9 and 10.

In each such group I computed the mean percentage reaction for each word in the series. For example :

TABLE XXII

Subject No. P1.

Reactions as percentages of their respective means.

Word:	Head	Green	Water	Sing	Dead
First test . .	86	10	0	76	257
Second test . .	0	0	65	0	588
Third test . .	0	0	0	0	145
Mean of 1, 2 and 3 .	29	3	22	25	330
Fourth test . .	0	0	0	0	254
Fifth test . .	55	0	0	0	276
Sixth test . · .	71	71	0	0	213
Mean of 4, 5 and 6 .	42	24	0	0	248
Mean of all tests .	35	14	11	12	289

I also calculated the mean percentage-reaction for all the tests, as shown above.

In order to ascertain what kind of effect is produced by using the means of two such groups of tests for each subject, instead of relying on a single pair of tests, and thus to gain some idea of how many tests it would be desirable to use in order to obtain reliable results in future work of this nature, I worked out the coefficients of correlation between the deflexions given by the first test and the second test respectively in the case of each subject. The correlations were :

TABLE XXIII

Correlation : first and second test for	P1	+·69
,, ,, ,,	P2	+·39
,, ,, ,,	P3	+·18
,, ,, ,,	P4	+·44
,, ,, ,,	P5	+·35
,, ,, ,,	P6	—·01
	Mean .	+·36

If these values are compared with those obtained from the correlation of the means of the groups it will be seen that the effect of taking the mean of several tests as a basis of calculation is greatly to increase the correlation and to eliminate the discrepancies between the performances of the same individual on different occasions.

I next calculated the coefficient of correlation between the means of the two groups (M1 and M2) for each subject and obtained the following correlation :

Table XXIV

Correlation:	first group (M1)	with second group (M2) for P1	+·98
,,	,, (M1)	,, (M2) ,, P2	+·72
,,	,, (M1)	,, (M2) ,, P3	+·70
,,	,, (M1)	,, (M2) ,, P4	+·60
,,	,, (M1)	,, (M2) ,, P5	+·68
,,	,, (M1)	,, (M2) ,, P6	+·42

The mean of these coefficients of correlations is +·68. If they be weighted in proportion to the number of observations on which each is based the weighted mean is +·685.

This value is important ; it is the mathematical expression of the extent to which an average subject agrees with himself, so to speak, over a period of the duration here involved (*i.e.* about three to four weeks).

The next step was to ascertain the extent to which subjects agree with each other. To ascertain this I worked out the coefficient of correlation between the mean percentage-reactions of all tests for each subject with every other subject. The resulting figures were :

Table XXV

Mean of P1 (all tests) with mean of		P2 (all tests)			+·19
,,	P1	,,	,,	P3	,,	—·02
,,	P1	,,	,,	P4	,,	+·12
,,	P1	,,	,,	P5	,,	—·01
,,	P1	,,	,,	P6	,,	+·02
,,	P2	,,	,,	P3	,,	+·15
,,	P2	,,	,,	P4	,,	+·19
,,	P2	,,	,,	P5	,,	+·18
,,	P2	,,	,,	P6	,,	+·01
,,	P3	,,	,,	P4	,,	+·46
,,	P3	,,	,,	P5	,,	+·14
,,	P3	,,	,,	P6	,,	—·24
,,	P4	,,	,,	P5	,,	+·23
,,	P4	,,	,,	P6	,,	—·04
,,	P5	,,	,,	P6	,,	—·13

The mean of these values is +·08. If they be weighted in proportion to the product of the number of observations on which each series correlated is based the weighted mean is +·09.

It will be noticed that with one exception (subject P3 with P4)[1] the correlation between any two subjects is very markedly lower than that between the two groups of any single individual subject. This is what we should expect on general grounds ; for, if we eliminate words of universal appeal from the list, the affective state evoked by any word in a given subject must be a product of that subject's personal experience : and the experience of every individual is unique.

In accordance with the ordinary laws of probability we should expect to find certain proportions of abnormally high and low values in each class of correlation (*i.e.* ' individuals with themselves ' and ' individuals with each other ') but the majority of values in each should approximate to the mean. We thus

---

[1] This is almost wholly due to two words, ' sad ' and ' waste,' which greatly excited both subjects : without these the figure would be about + ·09.

find the very high value of $+\cdot98$ for subject
P1 and the very low value of $+\cdot42$ for subject
P6, in the first class ; and the very high value
of $+\cdot46$ for subject P3 and P4.

If we had at our disposal a sufficiently large
number of values to give us the frequency
distributions of values in the two classes we
should doubtless obtain two overlapping curves
of which one would have its maximum at
approximately $+\cdot7$, the other at about $+\cdot1$. The
precise position of the maximum would depend,
inter alia, upon the number of words of universal
appeal which the list contained. If there were
none, the maximum of the curve corresponding
to the agreement between different individuals
would be exactly at o and it would, presumably,
be symmetrical, while that of the other curve
would be at about $+\cdot6$. Any increase in the
number of universally exciting words would
shift the maxima towards the right and, incident-
ally, bring them closer together ; for if the list
were composed exclusively of ' universal ' words
the element of individuality would, *ex hypothesi*,
be eliminated and the curves would coincide
with a maximum at $+1\cdot0$, becoming vertical
straight lines in the process.

From such curves it would be possible to
calculate the precise chance that a given coefficient of correlation between two series of
reactions of unknown origin arose from correlating the reactions of the same individual or of
two different individuals.

For practical purposes, however, such refine-
ments are unnecessary ; we may say with
considerable assurance that in general the correlation of individuals with themselves is about
$+\cdot60$ to $+\cdot70$, while the correlation between

different individuals is not likely to be greater than $+\cdot2$. The relevance of this conclusion to possible future investigations will be dealt with later.

It is necessary to give, at this stage, a few observations as to the experimental conditions under which this work was done and the probable reliability of the results obtained. I experienced a good deal of difficulty from the very cold weather which prevailed during part of the work and which was aggravated by the coal strike. I found that when subjects were cold and their skins dry and contracted they generally gave unsatisfactory reactions. Sometimes they refused to react at all and I was obliged to discontinue and to postpone several tests on this account. When they did react they generally gave very small deflexions with a distinct tendency towards an ' all-or-none ' type of reaction. That is to say, they would give long runs of very small deflexions, or of none at all, with what seemed to be disproportionately large deflexions for such few words as produced more than this minimal response. The effect of this is somewhat to increase the tendency of subjects to correlate highly with themselves and only slightly with each other, but I consider that this is at least discounted by the fact that such relatively unsatisfactory series of reactions appeared to be much more erratic than the more satisfactory series. Several of the tests in this experiment were as good as any I have observed and I received the strong impression that these ' conformed to type,' for any subject, much more closely than did the less good tests. That is to say, I anticipated large reactions on words which had previously excited the subject with far greater confidence when the test was one of first-class reliability than I did when it was not.

My opinion is that, in so far as the experimental conditions were adverse (and of course I never continued a test unless it was reasonably satisfactory), the effects very approximately cancelled each other, tending on the one hand to accentuate and on the other to diminish both the agreement of individuals with themselves and their lack of agreement with each other. This opinion is, of course, purely subjective, but it is based on a fairly extensive experience of using the galvanometer in conjunction with word-association tests and I have no doubt as to the reliability of the general results obtained.

Provided the tests are reasonably numerous and spread over a period of not more than a month, and that a suitable list of words is used, individuals will, in general, show a correlation with themselves of not less than $+\cdot6$ and, with each other, of not more than $+\cdot2$. (There will, of course, on the theory of probability, always be an occasional exception, as already pointed out.)

I may now pass to what I conceive to be the potential value of this method. I consider that it is likely to prove useful in the investigation of those phenomena of ' dissociation ' and ' multiple personality,' in which whole tracts of experience, so to speak, appear to become detached from, and to function independently of, the main mass of experience which determines the ' normal ' personality. There are, roughly speaking, two alternative views as to the kind of process which results in these conditions. On the one hand, they are regarded as no more than special cases of the general process of 'repression,' differing only from other instances of the same process in the extent and sharp delimitation of the mass of experiences repressed and in the intensity of the repression. On the other hand, it is suggested that some special process comes into play—a process distinct *sui generis* from anything operative in the normal mind—and that, as a result of this, the experiences concerned are actually, in some fashion, split off from the main mass and segregated, so to speak, into a water-tight compartment of their own. According to this view they are inactive, incapable of exerting any influence on mental-activity in the normal state, wholly autonomous and separated from the general mass of experience by an impassable barrier.

I, personally, incline very strongly to the former view, with which I suspect that most psychologists would agree ; but support of the other view, or of something closely resembling it, is not lacking from authoritative quarters.

This is the sort of point which might, in my opinion, be elucidated by the method which I have here described and in some measure tested. If it be conceded as a result of these experiments that it is possible to obtain a characteristic chart, so to speak, or at least to achieve a representative sampling, of a subject's mind by such means, it should be possible, in the light of this knowledge, to investigate the problem experimentally.

Consider a well-marked case of double personality in which the subject shows two alternative states, A and B, of which we will suppose that A is the normal, or relatively normal, state. If we test the subject in the *A* state on ten occasions, say, we shall obtain, if we use a reasonably large list of words, a set of mean reactions characteristic of the mental content determining that state. A similar testing of the *B* state will give us a set of reactions characteristic of the mental content of that state. If the correlation of these two sets of mean reactions proves to be of the same order as the correlation of an individual with himself—*i.e.* of the order of + ·65—we may conclude that the mental contents corresponding to and respectively determining the two states are essentially the same. But if the correlation is of the same order as that given by two different individuals—*i.e.* of the order of + ·1 or + ·2—we may conclude that the determining mental contents are different. To adopt the familiar, but valuable, analogy of the ' iceberg,' we should conclude in the first case that it is the same iceberg, but with a different area above the water and, in the second, that the iceberg has really been split into two parts.

As I have said, I anticipate that the former view would prove correct and this is to some extent supported by the work of Prince and Peterson in the ' Sally Beauchamp ' case described in the *Journal of Abnormal Psychology* for 1908.

These experimenters found that words which were emotionally significant to the patient in one state evoked a large psycho-galvanic reflex when presented to her in another, in spite of the fact that when in the latter state she was amnesic to the experiences which, in her first state, invested the words with their significance. The experiments were, however, few in number and of a relatively rough-and-ready nature. That is to say no attempt was made to show the agreement between the two states *quantitatively* and, even if this had been done, there was in existence no standard of comparison by which the extent of the agreement could be assessed.

Unfortunately, such clear-cut cases as this are rare, unless we include, as I think we should, those trance conditions commonly known as ' mediumistic.' These seem to me to deserve more attention from abnormal psychologists than they have yet received. To investigate such cases by the method described above would be very interesting and would almost certainly exhibit the trance ' controls '—to use the technical term—as no more than secondary personalities of the ' mediums ' concerned.

It would also be exceedingly interesting to apply the method to hypnotic subjects. Hypnosis is now believed by many authorities to depend essentially on an affective attitude of mind on the part of the subject towards the physician and it is at least possible that this might show itself in the reactions given by subjects who have been frequently hypnotised when compared with those who have not.

It is also possible that the reactions of a subject under hypnosis would differ appreciably from those of the same subject in his normal state, and if this were so we might obtain interesting light on the mental condition of a hypnotised subject.

It would also be interesting to ascertain whether it would be possible to abolish or to enhance the affective tone normally evoked by a stimulus-word by suggesting to the hypnotised subject that he should feel no emotion, or a great deal—as the case might be—when the word in question is called out.

Another point worth investigating would be the question of whether one could bring about any considerable redistribution of affective tone among the words of the list by suggesting to the subject that he is some person other than himself. It is well known that a hypnotised subject in a suitable condition will impersonate a suggested character with a fidelity and histrionic skill which are often remarkable. It would be interesting to ascertain whether such a suggested impersonation were accompanied by any radical redistribution of affective tone of anything like the same order as would necessarily be observed if the real individual impersonated were substituted for the hypnotised subject. Personally I do not anticipate that any such wholesale redistribution would take place, but some appreciable change is at least possible and, in any event, the question of the extent to which 'affect' can be displaced and redistributed by suggestion is a very interesting one, the answer to which would considerably enlarge our understanding of mental mechanisms and processes.

SUMMARY

(i) Individuals show marked and characteristic differences in the reactions they give to a suitably selected list of words.

(ii) Provided the mean values of several tests are taken and that these tests do not extend over too long a period individuals correlate with themselves much more highly than they do with each other.

(iii) The most probable values of the correlations of individuals with themselves and with each other may be taken as approximately $+\cdot65$ and $+\cdot15$ respectively, for a list of words of the kind here used. More extensive investigations could, if necessary, enable us to fix these values precisely, to determine the corresponding frequency distributions and thus to render future problems dealt with on these lines amenable to strict mathematical treatment.

(iv) These facts should enable us to determine whether certain tracts of experience ever become completely split off from the principal mass, and whether mental conditions which appear at first sight to differ *toto cælo* from each other are in reality determined by identically the same aggregate of experiences of which different aspects are thus expressed, or whether they proceed from aggregates so discrete and so independent of one another as to warrant our describing the resultant states as genuinely different personalities. They may also throw considerable light on various questions concerning the permanence and liability to disturbance of the affective tone concomitant to the experiences of an individual mind.

CHAPTER VI

EXPERIMENTS ON THE EFFECTS OF ALCOHOL

THE experiments described below were undertaken as a sequel to those dealt with in the preceding chapters, with the object of ascertaining how the affective tone of reactions and the complex-indicators accompanying them were modified by the action of alcohol. It was hoped that in this way some new light might be thrown on the psychological effects of the drug.

Although we often regard the psychological effects of alcohol as so familiar as to demand no special study or explanation, a few moments' thought will suffice to show that they are not nearly so straightforward as one might at first suppose.

On the one hand, it is a matter of common knowledge that under the influence of alcohol there is a tendency for people to react in an exaggerated fashion to inadequate stimuli ; they laugh hilariously, quarrel violently, weep copiously, all on the slenderest grounds. This suggests that they feel more acutely.

On the other hand, it is well-known that a man who is much worried, or for any reason unhappy, will often ' take to drink ' in order to alleviate his distress. This suggests that the effect of alcohol is to reduce intensity of feeling.

These few words are sufficient to show that the effects of alcohol are far from obvious, quite apart from the academic desirability of making an exact study of the psychological effects of all drugs.

External circumstances prevented the tests being performed on the same subjects as were examined in the course of the previous experiments. But, in any event, it would probably have been unwise to use the same subjects a second time, for their memories of the earlier tests might easily have affected their reactions and thus have rendered a true comparison impossible. Actually the subjects examined under alcohol were all of the same social and intellectual grades and of approximately the same ages as those previously considered, so it may be assumed that, without alcohol, they would have given, on the average, substantially identical results.

The experiments with alcohol were divided into two parts. The first series, performed on ten subjects, were undertaken primarily in order to ascertain whether the absolute magnitude of the psycho-galvanic reflex was increased or decreased by the administration of alcohol. It was not possible to determine this by comparison with the results of the previous experiments because the mean *absolute* magnitude of the reflex varies greatly among individuals, and from day to day in the same individual. It also varies with the size of the electrodes used, the strength of the salt-solution, the sensitivity of the electrical system,[1] etc.

[1] The apparatus used and procedure followed were the same as described in Chapter II.

In order to ascertain this point the following procedure was adopted : the original standard list of 100 words was divided into two lists of 50 words each. Of these 25 in each list were taken from the first half of the original list and 25 from the second half. Thus list A consisted of the words :

> Green, Sing, Ship, Make, Friend, Cold, Stalk, Village, Bring, Ink, Go, Carry, Bread, Tree, Yellow, Street, Bury, Salt, Habit, Pray, Silly, Despise, Finger, Paper, Wicked, Frog, Try, Hunger, Speak, Pencil, Marry, Nasty, Glass, Fight, Wine, Big, Doctor, Travel, Flower, Family, Name, Luck, Horse, Table, Afraid, Kiss, Choice, Bag, Happy, Wound,

of which the first 25 were taken from the first half of the original list.

Similarly, list B consisted of the words :

> Head, Water, Dead, Long, Woman, Cook, Ask, Dance, Pond, Sick, Proud, Angry, Needle, Swim, Blue, Lamp, Rich, Jump, Pity, Dress, Money, Book, War, Bird, Walk, White, Child, Sad, Plum, Home, Carrot, Give, Beat, Box, Old, Wait, Cow, Work, Brother, Love, Chair, Worry, Motor, Clean, Bed, State, Sheet, Evil, Divorce, Insult,

of which the first 25 were again taken from the first half of the original list.

The words in each of the two lists A and B were, moreover, so selected as to make the mean galvanometer deflexions for the two lists, obtained for the normal subjects previously examined, approximately equal. The mean for all the words in list A was 27·5 scale divisions and for list B 26·3.

The object in thus arranging the lists was to ensure that they should be as truly comparable as possible as regards galvanometer deflexions, apart from any influence which might be exerted by the administration of alcohol.

Each of the ten subjects selected for the first part of the experiment was tested, first in his normal state with one list and then, after the administration of alcohol, with the other list. The psycho-galvanic reflex and the reaction time were measured for each word and the ' reproduction test ' applied after each list. The dose of alcohol consisted of approximately a medium-sized wineglass of neat gin or whisky [1] and a period of from 10-20 minutes was allowed in each case in order to give the alcohol time to take effect. The precise size of the dose was varied slightly with individuals, less being given to abstainers than to those who were not. The object was rather to produce a uniform effect than to give a uniform dose and the subject was asked in each case whether he could distinctly feel the effects. If he could not do so, more alcohol was administered until he could.

In testing these subjects the order of the lists was reversed with alternate subjects so as to eliminate the small intrinsic differences between the lists. Thus, subject No. 1 was tested with list A before the alcohol and list B after ; No. 2 with list B before and list A after, etc.

It is safe to assume, I think, that if this procedure had been followed in every detail, with the exception of the alcohol, the mean deflexion of the list first used would, for the average of all subjects, be substantially identical with that of the list used second.

---

[1] Approximately equal to two ' large whiskies.'

THE MEASUREMENT OF EMOTION

The actual results were :

TABLE XXVI

Subject No.	Before alcohol Mean defln.	Mean RT	After alcohol Mean defln.	Mean RT
1	6·66	8·12	5·64	9·96
2	4·04	8·92	6·56	8·72
3	6·60	10·18	5·14	9·88
4	16·14	13·60	14·54	13·00
5	3·41	27·50	1·26	16·70
6	11·28	8·36	·46	9·80
7	25·56	9·56	24·74	10·10
8	49·10	12·82	30·82	15·82
9	34·80	10·96	28·00	11·92
10	33·32	10·30	34·50	9·12
Mean of means	19·09	12·32	15·17	11·50

It is clear that the effect of alcohol is to *reduce* the mean galvanometer deflexion. The ratio for the lists observed after alcohol to those observed before it is 15·17 : 19·09 = ·795.

This becomes still more striking if we apply, as we should, a correction for the variation in the mean resistance of each subject during the experiment.[1] The figures then become :

TABLE XXVII

Subject No.	Mean defln. before alcohol	Mean defln. after alcohol
1	8·66	6·20
2	5·84	4·75
3	2·38	1·72
4	7·10	5·23
5	1·33	·44
6	10·78	·37
7	14·93	9·14
8	12·27	6·47
9	8·01	4·76
10	49·98	41·40
Mean of means .	12·13	8·05

[1] See page 35.

The ratio in this case is 8·05 : 12·13 or ·665 : 1. (The mean of the individual ratios is ·592.) It will be noticed that in *every* case the corrected mean deflexion for the after-alcohol list is considerably less than that for the before-alcohol list.

It may, therefore, be regarded as established that the effect of alcohol is markedly to reduce the psycho-galvanic reflex as elicited by the word-association test.

The consideration of the effects observed with these subjects as regards force of association, reaction time and the reproduction test may be postponed until we deal with the results obtained in the course of the remainder of the experiments.

When this result concerning the absolute magnitude of the psycho-galvanic reflex had been obtained, I no longer felt it necessary to employ the comparative method described above with each individual subject. Accordingly, I resorted to the use of my complete original list, with which I tested each of a further twenty subjects who were given a dose of alcohol (of the size and nature described above) before starting the test.

The general results are summarised in the following table :

TABLE XXVIII

Subject No.	Mean RT	Mean GD	Mean GD (corrected)	Failures in reproduction %
11	9·81	25·26	58·09	17
12	11·61	14·34	30·11	33
13	17·21	30·40	63·84	52
14	10·60	13·55	25·27	22
15	10·28	12·93	35·56	28
16	13·38	·95	6·65	41
17	9·75	11·17	44·68	13
18	8·72	17·48	58·56	25
19	18·55	13·63	53·16	49
20	10·12	9·83	20·64	19
21	9·32	1·80	18·00	24
22	10·78	4·92	68·88	24
23	9·42	18·02	23·97	25
24	9·69	8·50	16·15	27
25	10·95	9·40	21·62	15
26	8·73	32·45	58·41	27
27	9·59	21·09	51·67	30
28	14·28	5·53	12·17	38
29	10·01	13·09	45·81	31
30	9·70	19·83	56·52	19
Means .	11·12		33·49	27·95
Corresponding means for normal subjects	11·22	..	..	26·90

When it is remembered that the galvanometer deflexions of these subjects are not directly comparable with those of normal subjects (for the reasons already given) and that in the case of the latter the mean reaction time and mean percentage of failures in reproduction are 11·22 and 26·90 respectively, it is clear that these figures are not very helpful as they stand. The data require much more elaborate analysis before useful results can be obtained from them.[1] Such very slight differences as there were, however (1% decrease in reaction time and 4% in mean number of failures in reproduction),

[1] In the course of this detailed analysis I shall pay considerably more attention to galvanometer deflexions than to reaction times, for, as I have shown above, the former is a far more delicate measure of affective tone.

suggest a diminution rather than an increase in emotional activity.

The first point with which I dealt was that of the variability of the reactions given by ' alcoholic ' as compared with normal subjects. It has always seemed to me that this quality —measured by the ' mean variation ' or more reliably by the ' coefficient of variation ' is calculated to give a reasonably good measure of the ' emotivity ' of a subject. The term ' emotivity ' is admittedly difficult to define with precision although most of us probably attach some sort of meaning to the word. But I think it is clear that a subject who reacts in very different degrees to stimuli of differing intensities may fairly be said to possess a higher ' emotivity ' than one who maintains a uniform dead level of response.[1] The affective mechanisms of the latter would appear to be imperfectly developed, his emotional life poor in quality, his capacity for feeling, excitement and interest deficient ; while the former would be more responsive, capable of a richer emotional experience and altogether less inert.

In order, therefore, to compare alcoholic with normal subjects in this respect I computed the mean variation and the coefficient of variation [2] for the mean reactions elicited by the words of the list for the two classes in question. The results were :

---

[1] This applies even if the absolute mean magnitude of the reactions is large, for this may be due to low initial skin resistance or to other causes. Cf. p. 35.

[2] Mean variation $=\dfrac{\Sigma \delta}{n \times M}$ where δ is the difference of any variates from the mean (M) and n is the number of variates : Coefficient of Variation is $\sqrt{\dfrac{\Sigma \delta^2}{n \times M}}$.

TABLE XXIX

Mean variation :	Normal subjects	0·25
,, ,,	Alcoholic ,, ...	0·22
Coefficient of variation :	Normal ,, ...	0·345
,, ,,	Alcoholic ,, ...	0·28

In each case the variability of alcoholic subjects is seen to be appreciably less than that of normal subjects and it is worth noting that the coefficient of variation (which is the more reliable measure) shows the difference more strongly than does the mean variation.

As a check on this I calculated the coefficients of variation of a number of alcoholic and normal subjects individually. For this purpose I selected my six 'best' normal subjects—that is to say those six subjects who had most impressed me by the smoothness, reliability and regularity of their reactions. This impression of reliability was to a great extent inversely proportional to the erraticness of the subjects examined and the six subjects selected are, therefore, likely to have coefficients of variation considerably *below* the average for normal persons.

The values obtained were :

TABLE XXX

Subject No.	Coefficient of Variation
1	·503
2	·911
26	·579
28	1·440
33	·544
48	1·260
Mean .	·873

From my alcoholic subjects I took the first

six of those who did the whole test under the influence of alcohol.

The results were :

TABLE XXXI

Subject No.	Coefficient of Variation
11	·438
12	·597
13	·536
14	·360
15	·324
16	·804
Mean .	·510

No. 16 is fairly obviously a ' freak.' The values for the next three are ·452, ·729, ·793. The mean for the first nine (including No. 16) is ·56 ; if No. 16 is excluded the value for the first six (viz. 11, 12, 13, 14, 15 and 17) is ·45.

It is clear, therefore, that the coefficient of variation is saliently less for alcoholic than for normal persons.

That is to say, the effect of alcohol is to diminish emotivity *on the whole*.[1]

The next step was to classify the reactions obtained from the alcoholic subjects according to their ' indicator classes ' (see Chapter III).

The results were :

Class	O	T	G	R	TG	TR	GR	TGR	Total
No. of reactions	706	294	408	153	368	139	116	238	2422
% of total	29·1	12·1	16·8	6·3	15·3	5·8	4·8	9·8	100

[1] I italicise these words because, as will be seen later, there appears to be a kind of *redistribution* of emotional activity, which results in certain strongly affective reactions being more numerous in spite of the general emotivity being lowered.

The corresponding figures for normal subjects are :

Class	O	T	G	R	TG	TR	GR	TGR	Total
No. of reactions	480	255	307	129	239	119	105	107	1741
% of total	27·6	14·7	17·6	7·4	13·7	6·8	6·0	6·2	100

The ratios $\left\{\dfrac{\text{alcoholic subjects}}{\text{normal subjects}}\right\}$ of the percentages are :

Class	O	T	G	R	TG	TR	GR	TGR
Ratio	1·06	·82	·95	·85	1·12	·85	·80	1·58

These figures are exceedingly curious. The most noticeable thing is the marked increase in the class TGR—the class which is accompanied by the most intense degree of negative tone. Next comes TG, the class accompanied by the most intense degree of positive tone. Third in order is class O composed of indifferent words. These three gain, under alcohol, at the expense of the classes corresponding to reactions accompanied by only a moderate degree of tone. Thus if, as seems reasonably legitimate, we classify reactions as (i) ' highly toned ' (consisting of classes TG and TGR) ; (ii) ' moderately toned ' (classes T, G, R, TR and GR) ; and (iii) ' untoned ' (class O), we have :

Ratios of percentages of reactions among alcoholic as compared with normal subjects :

(i) Highly toned reactions . . . . 1·26
(ii) Moderately toned reactions . . . ·87
(iii) Untoned reactions . . . . 1·05

Or if, as may be thought more correct in the light of the observations on pp. 66-68, we include class T among the 'untoned' reactions, we have :

(i) Highly toned reactions .	.	.	1·26
(ii) Moderately toned reactions	.	.	·89
(iii) Untoned reactions	.	.	·98

In either case it is clear that highly toned reactions have considerably gained at the expense of the moderately toned, while in the first case the neutral or untoned reactions have also slightly increased and in the second slightly diminished.

The status of class ' T ' as a true ' neutral ' or untoned class has always been rather doubtful (see pp. 65-68) and I am not sure whether, in this context, the first or the second of the two modes of classification used above is the more correct. The point is, however, of minimal importance and we may content ourselves with saying that the proportion of neutral reactions is substantially unchanged.

The really important point is the gain in highly toned reactions and the loss in moderately toned, and this is unmistakable in each case.

In other words, it is clear that under the influence of alcohol *reactions tend towards an ' all-or-none ' character*.

In order to test still further the conclusions already reached I next proceeded to classify the reactions obtained according to the verbal form of the association. I therefore computed the numbers of associations falling in the various classes described in Chapter IV.

The results are shown in Table XXXII, which also shows the corresponding figure for normal subjects :

TABLE XXXII

	Alcoholic subjects Class	No.	%	The corresponding figures for normal subjects are : No.	%	Ratio of the % are :
Inner associations	I	437	17·9	287	17·4	1·04
	II (b)	52	2·1	75	4·5	·47
	II (e)	84	3·3	50	3·0	1·17
	III	80	3·5	57	3·4	·97
	VII	109	4·5	86	5·2	·86
	Total	762	31·3	555	33·5	·93
Outer associations	II (a)	319	13·0	229	13·8	·94
	II (c)	48	2·0	39	2·4	·83
	II (d)	199	8·2	141	8·5	·97
	IV	310	12·6	264	14·8	·85
	V	244	10·0	104	6·3	1·57
	VI (a)	481	19·6	285	17·2	1·14
	VI (b)	48	2·0	37	2·2	·91
	VI (c)	25	1·3	22	1·3	1·00
	Total	1674	68·7	1121	66·5	1·03
	Grand total	2436	100	1676	100	

I have no doubt that one could draw various interesting conclusions from a detailed consideration of the gains and losses of these various classes under the influence of alcohol. But I do not think that such conclusions would be sufficiently reliable to justify the undertaking. The verbal form of the association is much more under voluntary and conscious control than is the reaction time, while the galvanometer deflexion is, of course, not under control at all. Consequently, although the verbal form is a useful guide where broad differences are in question, I would not care to rely upon it in detail when we are concerned only with delicate *differential* effects, such as are produced in normal persons by the administration of a relatively small dose of alcohol.

For our present purpose, therefore, it is sufficient to note that the proportion of ' inner ' associations is diminished, while that of ' outer ' associations is increased.

In order to ascertain whether this difference is likely to be significant, I have applied the method described in Appendix III to the percentages of inner associations given by normal (33·5%) and alcoholic (31·3%) subjects respectively. The figures are :

	Normal subjects	Alcoholic subjects
Root mean square of deviation of percentages of inner associations from mean percentage .	6·85	6·29
Number of subjects . . .	18	20
Probable error . . .	± 1·09	± ·95
Value of ' p '	1·03	
Chance of the observed difference being accidental . . .	·152	

That is to say, the chances are about 5·6 to 1 in favour of this difference being a *bona fide* effect due to the influence of alcohol.

This piece of evidence is of some slight importance because it reduces the chance that the observed decrease in the psycho-galvanic reflex [1] is due to direct physiological causes and makes it almost certain that it is, partially at least, a genuinely psychological phenomenon.

The evidence then consists of the following items :

(i) The absolute mean magnitude of the psycho-galvanic reflex is diminished.
(ii) The variability of the reflex is also diminished.
(iii) The proportion of inner associations is smaller.
(iv) The proportion of highly toned reactions is increased at the expense of the moderately toned.

[1] Page 35.

(v) Possibly the proportion of neutral reactions is slightly increased—*i.e.* the threshold of response is slightly raised—but this is doubtful.

This being so, we may describe the effects of alcohol as two in number :

(i) There is a general lowering of emotivity.
(ii) *The type of reaction tends to regress towards a more ' all-or-none ' or protopathic type.*

This seems to me to be extremely interesting. It has often been suggested—on general grounds —that a person under the influence of alcohol approximates to a more primitive type, as indeed is often obvious from his behaviour. But here we have concrete experimental evidence, based solely on measurement, that this is actually the case. This appears to me to harmonise with the point of view (developed, for example, by Dr Rivers in his *Instinct and the Unconscious*), which stresses the gradual transition from protopathic to epicritic modes of reaction, on the psychological in addition to the physiological levels, as organisms rise in the evolutionary scale.

In the light of this view we can reconcile the paradox outlined on page 124, by saying that under the influence of alcohol a person is, on the whole, slightly more inert, in the sense that many stimuli produce a smaller effect in him than in the normal person ; but that if the stimuli once surpass a certain value the result in behaviour tends to become extreme. This accords well both with my experimental results and the observed behaviour of partially intoxicated individuals.

It is clear from the foregoing that the technique developed in these pages is competent to throw considerable light on the psychological effects of drugs. Further experiments with larger doses of alcohol would be valuable, but still more so would be investigations of other drugs, such as opium, cocaine, heroin, strychnine, amyl nitrite, Indian hemp or bhang. In particular, it would be interesting to ascertain what drugs, if any, produce an opposite effect to that of alcohol and lead to a *less* protopathic mode of reaction, of a type, that is to say, corresponding to a supernormal instead of a subnormal level of evolution. Moreover, it would be of the utmost interest and importance to attempt to correlate these psychological effects with the known physiological effects of the drugs. In this way we could fairly hope greatly to increase our knowledge of the physical correlates of mental processes.

SUMMARY

(i) The effect of alcohol is to reduce the absolute magnitude of the psycho-galvanic reflex. This is probably partly due to direct physiological causes, but is also partially of psychological origin.

(ii) The variability of the reflex is reduced.

(iii) The proportion of inner associations is smaller.

(iv) The proportion of highly toned reactions is increased at the expense of the *moderately* toned : the proportion of *untoned* remains substantially unchanged.

(v) Thus it is shown experimentally that, in addition to a slight all-round raising of the threshold of emotional response and a tendency to mistrust, the effect of alcohol is to cause a regression to a more primitive, all-or-none or protopathic type of reaction.

CHAPTER VII

THE THEORY OF AFFECTIVE TONE

WITH the last chapter I concluded my account of my experimental work and I will now return to the consideration of some theoretical aspects of affective tone which I touched on in my first chapter.

My principal object is to explain more fully, and to justify as far as possible, the use of the terms ' positive ' and ' negative ' affective tone, which I have used so freely in this book. I believe that these concepts are likely to prove of value in the development of psychological theory and I am very anxious that there should be no doubt whatever as to their intended scope and meaning.

It is now generally recognised that every mental state possesses some kind of emotional quality, and it is a common and convenient practice to speak of it in this respect as having ' affective tone.'

The number of varieties of tone which we distinguish is simply a matter of convenience and there is no fundamental objection to our using different systems of classification on different occasions according to the purpose of our investigation.

Thus Dr Myers, speaking at the British Association in 1921, distinguished four varieties, namely, those characterised by (a) strain, and (b) relaxation in response to a favourable situation, and by (c) strain, and (d) relaxation in response to one unfavourable.

This is a perfectly good and legitimate classification whenever, and so long as, the discussion of any problem is facilitated thereby. But it is obviously not the only possible one, although it has the great merit of defining its categories in fairly unambiguous terms and of affording obvious opportunities of correlating any psychological conclusions deduced from it with physiological and biological factors.

The value of any classification of varieties of affective tone must depend solely on the use that is to be made of it and in this chapter I propose to contend that the concepts of ' positive ' and ' negative ' tone, defined as I have defined them, are of fundamental utility.

In view of what I have just written it is clear that I must start by stating what I conceive to be the object of any such classification and this is equivalent to a statement of the whole object of psychological investigation.

I do not think it will be denied that this is to study and elucidate the mechanism responsible for mental activity and I hold, therefore, that no account of affective tone is of any value unless, and except in so far as, it is considered and explained in its capacity as a part of that mechanism.

Mental activity consists in a succession of mental states, or rather in a continuous flux of which a mental state is an instantaneous section, and I hold the view that any mental state can be described in terms of two irreducibles which, provisionally, I call Attention and Ideas or Systems of Ideas. I am well aware that there are many difficulties latent in these terms, especially in the latter, but it is not easy to find any satisfactory substitute. I have previously spoken of 'presentations' and 'groups of presentations,' but if it were not for the controversies which centre round the problem of 'imageless thought' and certain difficulties connected with perception, I should be disposed to use the word 'images' in preference to either of the two alternatives given above, and in dealing with such processes as Memory, Dream, Phantasy and Hallucination it is clearly adequate and free from ambiguity. But, on the whole, I prefer, at present, to keep to 'presentations,' 'groups of presentations,' or, more generally, 'ideas.'

Psychology, then, consists primarily in the study of the incidence of attention upon ideas, or—to paraphrase this slightly—the accession of ideas to consciousness ; and so far as psychologists are concerned with the working of the individual mind as actually encountered their business is to elucidate the laws which determine this incidence.

The foregoing must not be taken as implying that the psychologist is not concerned with unconscious processes and factors ; they are, on the contrary, of supreme importance. But this importance is derived solely from their capacity as causal determinants of the kinds of mental state referred to above, and if it were not for the latter we should never have been led to study them. If the content of the Unconscious exerted no influence on that of the Conscious we should know nothing of it and care less ; we can only deal, in the first instance and at first hand, with 'end-products.' Everything else is a matter of inference, not direct experience.

In dream, for example, the manifest content is determined by all manner of unconscious factors, but psychologists would have remained ignorant of, and indifferent to them but for the necessity of explaining and interpreting that manifest content.

It is clear, I think, that from this point of view it is useless to begin by talking of pleasant and unpleasant emotion, of sexual emotion, of emotions of rage, pain, grief, shame, anxiety or joy. Such a classification may be convenient for certain purposes but the categories are very vague, the emotions classified are often of a mixed nature and the terms used have no reference to the influence which these emotions exert on the accession to consciousness of the ideas which they accompany.

As already indicated in my first chapter, I think it would be better not to use the terms 'emotion' and 'affective tone' as interchangeable, but rather to reserve the former for discussion of 'the emotions,' as exemplified above, and to use only the latter when dealing with the elementary mechanisms of mental activity. For there are only two possible modes in which the affective tone concomitant to an idea can affect attention—only two ways in which the accession of that idea to consciousness can be influenced : attention may be attracted or repelled, the accession may be promoted or impeded, but no third effect is conceivable. Hence, for the student of mental processes as such, the classification of emotions as painful, pleasant, grievous, shameful, sexual, anxious, joyous and so forth is valueless, for such terms do not imply which of these effects is exerted by the emotions to which they refer.

This point of view may be restated less formally, but perhaps more effectively, as follows : A man dreams and certain assemblages of presentations, ideas, images—call them what you will—succeed one another in his mind ; he remembers or imagines and a similar process takes place ; he acts, and again his field of consciousness is filled with certain images or presentations albeit of a different kind. As a student of individual psychology my business is to explain how and why his attention is incident upon just those particular images or presentations ; I must ask myself why they and not others are present in his field of consciousness, and a knowledge of the origin and properties of affective tone interests me only in so far as it enables me to answer that question.

The foregoing should make it clear why I have proposed to use the terms ' positive ' and ' negative ' when speaking of affective tone rather than ' pleasant ' and ' unpleasant ' or any similar antithesis. The former terms probably do, as a matter of fact, correspond fairly closely to the latter and represent qualities genetically derived from them, but there are certainly many exceptions to the correspondence and an account of affective tone based on the antithesis of pleasant and unpleasant will not take us very far in our attempt to understand the part it plays in mental processes. If ' pleasantly ' toned ideas always reached the field of consciousness and ' unpleasant ' ones always failed to do so, the distinction would be helpful ; but this is not the case, and if we were to start on this basis there would come a time, sooner or later, when we should be forced to inquire into the circumstances in which unpleasant ideas force their way into consciousness. This inquiry is fundamental and it seems to me that the best course is to start by postulating two opposite varieties of affective tone to be defined by their effects in this all-important respect.

If it be objected that this postulation is unjustified and that perhaps there are not two opposite kinds of tone after all, I would answer, first, that this view is fully in accord with modern psychological thought in general and, second, that my experimental results adequately support it. Throughout that field of psychology, which may roughly be described as psycho-analytical, we find statements to the effect that certain ideas are ' repressed,' or admitted to consciousness only in a disguised form, on account of the ' painful,' ' conflicting ' or ' disagreeable ' tone which would be produced by their uncensored presence. Similarly, those ideas are represented as readily admitted to consciousness which, because they fulfil a wish, or for other reasons, are productive of ' pleasant ' tone.

On the experimental side I have shown that especial intensity of affective tone, as measured by the psycho-galvanic reflex, may influence the accession to consciousness of the ideas which it accompanies in two diametrically opposite ways. It may facilitate this accession or it may impede it and this can only be explained intelligibly by saying that, so far as accession to consciousness is concerned, there are two kinds of affective tone possessed of opposite properties. This conclusion can only be evaded by denying that the psycho-galvanic reflex indicates affective tone at all and I do not think that any psychologist acquainted with the phenomenon is likely to do this.

Having thus, as I hope, cleared the ground and left no doubt as to my *point de départ* I can proceed to the main part of the discussion.

One of the first points which demands consideration is the question of whether affective tone is to be regarded as being of the nature of an *attribute* of the ideas which it accompanies, in the same sort of way as colour or density are attributes of material objects. It is not uncommon to hear psychologists speak of ' affect ' almost as if it were a substance which sticks to ideas and could, if only we were clever enough, be detached and put in a bottle. They do not, of course, really mean to suggest anything so ridiculous as this ; but I think they do mean to suggest that ' affect ' is either a separate entity *sui generis,* or else an attribute inseparable from ideas and not wholly dependent on the context of the latter.

As against this I would support the view that affective tone proceeds essentially from *relations* between different ideas or systems of ideas and is in no sense an attribute of them. This view has at least two merits: in the first place, it is simpler than the alternative ; for, in any event, we must postulate ideas and relations between them and if we can explain affective tone in terms of these postulates there is nothing to be gained—but something to be lost—by regarding it as a distinct entity *sui generis* and, as such, an additional ' irreducible.' Secondly, it can scarcely be denied that the affective tone of an idea is, in some measure at least, a function of its context ; if not of its immediate context, then of its

context in past experience. That the idea of
yellow, say, should arouse intense affective tone
in *A* and none at all in *B* can scarcely be explained otherwise than by supposing differences
of emotional significance between the situations
in which it has figured for the two persons concerned.

We may now consider the kinds of relation
between ideas, or systems thereof, which lead
to the two opposite varieties of tone.

As a first approximation I suggest that the
matter is one of conflict or harmony. Whenever a situation tends to call up, by association,
groups of incompatible and opposed ideas, there
results one variety of affective tone, while, if
they are compatible and reinforce one another,
the other variety of tone is produced.

But this conception of conflict and harmony
requires further elucidation. To say that those
ideas conflict which are ' incompatible ' does not,
of itself, take us very far. For it seems clear
that there are many ideas, or groups of ideas,
which might fairly be called incompatible but
which could not reasonably be regarded as
conflicting and whose juxtaposition in the field
of consciousness is certainly not productive of
affective tone. Thus, if I am asked " Where is
John ? " and I am not sure whether he is in
Cambridge or not, there may well be present
within my field of consciousness two groups of
ideas corresponding to ' John-in-Cambridge '
and ' John-not-in-Cambridge ' respectively. But
although these two groups of ideas are logically
incompatible—since John cannot both be in
Cambridge and not be in Cambridge—their
incompatibility will not, of itself, produce any
affective state in my mind. Merely formal

incompatibility is clearly not the characteristic of that relationship of conflict which results in one of the two varieties of affective tone (*i.e.* negative tone).

I suggest that conflict arises only when, and in so far as, the systems of ideas concerned tend towards opposing or incompatible organic adjustments or reactions. To express this slightly differently, I might say that affective tone results from the conflict or harmony of simultaneously evoked *wishes* or ' wish-tendencies.' [1] This may seem somewhat far-fetched, but I do not think that it is really so. A more acceptable way of putting it, perhaps, would be to say that the conflict or harmony is between different conative elements in the total mental state, and I doubt whether any psychologist would maintain that any mental state is wholly devoid of conative elements. Much depends on what we understand by the word ' wish,' and in this matter I share the view of Holt, who says :

> " It (the wish) is a course of action which the body takes, or is prepared (by motor set) to take with regard to objects, relations, or events in the environment. The prophetic quality of thought which makes it seem that thought is the hidden and inner secret of conduct is the preceding labile interplay of motor settings which goes on almost constantly, and which differs from overt conduct in that the energy involved is too small to produce gross bodily movements." [2]

[1] At any rate it is the conflict between such wish-tendencies that produces negative tone. Positive tone may, perhaps, not always require two systems for its production.

[2] *The Freudian Wish*, p. 94.

The view I have suggested is easy enough to accept if we consider an artificially simple case in which a situation may evoke by the usual processes of association and innate physiological mechanisms ideas antecedent to mutually exclusive reactions—groups of motor presentations, in fact, which, if attended to, would lead to incompatible actions. But it is admittedly harder to grasp in the case of mental processes which, superficially at least, appear to be purely 'intellectual' and to have nothing whatever to do with action of any kind.

As a matter of fact I doubt whether any mental process can properly be considered as wholly divorced from prospective action, although it may not be easy in any given case to identify the particular actions which it indirectly foreshadows. But, however indirect the connexion may be, however many links in the chain may intervene between action and the passing thought, it must be conceded, I think, that the latter occurs only by virtue of its relevance to and associations with the former. The idea that a man thinks merely for the sake of thinking is one which I find it impossible to entertain ; he thinks as a prelude to action, as a necessary antecedent to those reactions and adjustments to his environment, the necessity for which constitutes, strictly speaking, the sole *raison d'être* for mental processes of any kind.

This also is well expressed by Holt :

" Thought is latent course of action with regard to environment (*i.e.* is motor setting) . . . but . . . Will is also course of action with regard to environment, so that the

only difference between thought and voli-
tion is one of the intensity of nerve impulse
which plays through the sensori-motor arcs
—a difference of minimal importance for
psychology." [1]

It must never be forgotten that psychology
is one of the biological sciences and that the
whole of biological science may be described
as the story of the adaptation of organisms
to their environment. This necessity for adaptation is the driving-power, so to speak, responsible for every form of vital activity and is the
cardinal principle which must never be lost
sight of throughout the study of any biological
problem. (If exception be taken to my use of
the phrase ' driving-power,' I would merely
point out that organisms which behave *as if*
this were the case—no matter what may be
the real reason for their behaviour—have a
greater chance of surviving than those which
do not. This has led to the elimination of
the latter in favour of the former and the existing state of affairs is, consequently, prag-
matically indistinguishable from that which is
implied in the preceding sentences.)

To this principle the amœba in its pond and
so relatively complex and sensitive an organism
as a modern politician are alike subservient.
Each reacts in such a way as to adapt himself
as perfectly as possible to his environment,
no matter whether the changes in the latter
are in respect of such simple matters as tempera-
ture, pressure or salinity or the more subtle
influences of Ethical beliefs and Voting power.

The points I wish to make are that, so soon

[1] *The Freudian Wish*, p. 98.

150

as we adopt a broad biological standpoint, mental processes must be regarded as simply and solely a part of the total mechanism whereby the adaptation of the organism to its environment is secured ; that this process of adaptation must, in the last analysis, resolve itself into organic adjustments of some kind ; and that all mental states must, therefore, be inextricably bound up with conative tendencies, wishes, and those varieties of presentation—motor presentations to wit—attention to which is productive of adaptative action.[1]

I need hardly say that I use the term ' environment ' in the widest possible sense to include all forces and factors, of whatever nature, which may in any way influence the organism. I also realise that inasmuch as individuals differ from one another, so the degree of their adaptation to externally identical environments will also differ. But whether the individual's adaptation be effected by changing the environment or by changing itself, it must equally proceed from reactions and organic adjustments of one kind or another.

To revert : affective tone, in my view, may be said to proceed from the simultaneous evocation of different systems of ideas containing, *inter alia*, conative elements or wish-tendencies appropriate to the real situation corresponding to the idea evoked. These involve subliminal [2] innervations of the physiological mechanisms which would be concerned in the reaction. If these reactions and adjustments are incom-

---

[1] Cf. Ward, *Psychological Principles*, Chapter II, etc.

[2] I use the word ' subliminal ' to denote innervations too weak to result in overt actions—what Holt calls " gross bodily movement."

patible a conflict of a physiological nature takes place, an inhibition or blocking occurs and endosomatic sensations are thereby generated which, when perceived, give rise to one variety of affective tone. (I shall deal with the other variety shortly.)

This close connexion of thought with potential action is readily appreciated if we consider certain simple cases of it. To take an extreme case, we all know how we tend instinctively to clench our fists if we are angered, and a similar but fainter innervation can often be traced in other cases. If, for example, I imagine myself dancing, I can identify certain faint kinæsthetic sensations proceeding from the muscles of my legs and trunk, as well as the appropriate visual and auditory images. The connexion is admittedly far less obvious in the case of more ' abstract ' thinking ; but inasmuch as all mental processes are ultimately directed towards adaptative adjustment of some kind, it seems probable that the same process is always at work, though in a less direct and palpable way.

Consider, for example, what happens if I receive a telegram stating that " Jones is dead." If Jones is in any way significant to me, if he plays any part in my life at all, it is on account of certain reactions of my own towards situations in which he is an element. Apart from those situations and the reactions which they provoke he would be nothing at all to me, and whenever the idea of Jones is present to my mind there must be present also, in some measure, the presentations corresponding to those situations and those reactions. My distress (or elation) at the demise of Jones proceeds, it would appear, from the prospective inhibition or nullification of those reactions.

Hitherto, I have laid more stress on the causes which lead to the production of that variety of affective tone which corresponds to conflict (negative tone) than to the other variety. I have done this because it is fairly easy to understand, in principle at least, how the simultaneous evocation of systems of ideas containing conative tendencies towards incompatible reactions may lead to nervous impulses competing, so to speak, for mutually exclusive efferent paths and, by their reciprocal inhibition or blocking, occasioning an endosomatic disturbance, which in turn would originate afferent impulses appreciated as affective tone. It is not quite so easy to imagine how the other variety of tone (positive) comes about, but I think it is quite practicable to advance reasonable suggestions with regard to it. I might, of course, content myself with claiming that if conflict and inhibition are responsible for one variety of tone, then it is likely that harmony and reinforcement will produce the other variety. In these particular circumstances I think that such a course would be legitimate, but it is obviously open to criticism on logical grounds.

Moreover, although I have suggested that conative tendencies and their concomitant subliminal innervations are productive of both kinds of tone, I do not consider that the mechanism responsible for this effect is precisely the same in the case of positive tone as that described above in considering negative tone. It is difficult to imagine how innervations which reinforce one another could produce a recoil, so to speak, of nervous energy in the form of afferent impulses in the way which seems comprehensible enough in cases when there is blocking and inhibition.

One possible view would be that positive tone results from a relaxation of the tension which constitutes what we call our ' normal ' state—the state, that is, in which we are not conscious of any marked affective tone of either kind. It could plausibly be maintained, I think, that this state is not one of *absolute* but of *relative* absence of conflict. In every situation there are, I conceive, elements calculated to provoke, however faintly, many different kinds of organic adjustment or reaction. That these reactions do not become overt means simply that they are inhibited, and if inhibited then there must result the state of affairs productive of negative tone as above described. Our unconsciousness of this is precisely paralleled by our unconsciousness of normal tone in the skeletal muscles or of a long-continued stimulus to which we have become habituated. But we all know that, in the latter case, cessation of the stimulus is at once noticed. Similarly, it may be suggested that so soon as the presentations corresponding to these inhibited reactions are succeeded in consciousness by others corresponding to a reaction against which no inhibiting forces are opposed—for whatever reasons this reaction may be evoked—this normal state of tension or negative tone vanishes, its cessation is perceived and this perception constitutes the other variety of tone. According to this view the tone consequent upon the relaxation of the antecedent tension would be in the nature of a

' contrast effect ' and its intensity would increase in proportion to that of the tension relaxed. This accords with the known character of the feeling of ' relief ' which accompanies the cessation of acute conflict.[1]

I do not wish to attach any considerable weight to this suggestion, but I think it not impossible that the processes in question may play some part in the production of affective tone. In particular the probability that the absence of inhibition and conflict in the normal state is only relative seems to me to be worth bearing in mind, especially in view of its close resemblance to, and possible connexion with, the phenomena of normal skeletal tone ; for these last constitute an additional link between the psychological and physiological aspects of the questions involved.

The alternative view of the origin of that variety of affective tone which results from the evocation of systems of ideas tending to produce compatible reactions may be conveniently deferred until I have made a short digression on the subject of Pain and Pleasure as such.

So far I have concerned myself solely with the affective tone which accompanies the accession of systems of ideas to consciousness. But experience indicates that affective tone may result from circumstances in which the ideas present to consciousness play no apparent part at all. There can be no doubt that, in general, the sensation of Pain—produced by the stimulation of the appropriate receptors— is negatively toned, but it is not at first sight clear how this tone can be said to arise from the conflict of incompatible conative tendencies.

[1] Compare Dr Myers' classification of affective tone cited above.

Mutatis mutandis the same applies to the positive tone which normally accompanies the enjoyment of any sensuous pleasure.

There are two explanations which might be adopted in order to bring these phenomena into line with the views expressed above. At first sight the simplest is to regard pain-sensations (and their opposites) as constituting merely a sub-division of that class of sensations, previously referred to, whose perception gives rise to affective tone. According to this view the affective tone arising from pain, for instance, would only differ from that occasioned by the evocation of conflicting ideas by the fact that the former can be aroused by the direct stimulation of receptors by external influences, while the latter is due to the reciprocal inhibition of nervous impulses and consequent endosomatic disturbance. The position could then be stated as follows :

There is a class of sensations whose presence in consciousness constitutes the affective tone of mental states ; of these some produce one variety of tone while others produce the opposite. These two sub-classes may further be roughly divided into sensations produced by the stimulation of definite receptors and those which are not : the latter are occasioned by processes of inhibition or the reverse within the body itself.

But this view is open to criticism on the ground that our perception of pain, for example, is not identical with the affective tone concomitant to it ; two distinct things seem to be involved, and in certain cases the affective tone accompanying sensations of pain may be definitely positive.

I incline, therefore, to the alternative view

which regards the affective tone accompanying pain as determined by causes precisely similar to those responsible for the tone produced by the conflict of opposed ideas ; that is to say, by the blocking of innervations antecedent to reactions.

The sensation of pain invariably tends to produce an immediate and well-marked reaction of a nature calculated to remove the affected part from the vicinity of the cause of the pain. I suggest that the affective tone of a mental state which includes pain-sensations is determined by the obstruction, if any, which this reaction encounters. In the limiting case where there is no obstruction of any kind and where, consequently, the reaction is carried out and the cessation of pain secured the instant the sensation is perceived, there will be no affective tone ; but there is, in practice, always some delay and consequently some affective tone. This, of course, is markedly the case when, as a result of injury to tissues or for other reasons, there is no reaction which can bring alleviation.

If a blister has been raised on my hand by burning, the pain persists and although the reaction to pain in that case may consist in a withdrawal of the hand in a perfectly well determined manner, this reaction must be inhibited since it cannot, for external reasons, be continued indefinitely ; hence the negative affective tone concomitant to the condition, as distinct from the sensation of pain as such.

Similar considerations may perhaps be applied to the affective tone aroused by the direct stimulation of those receptors which give rise to feelings of sensuous pleasure.

In the case of negative tone due to the evocation of ideas, the endosomatic disturbances are set up, as already described, by the reciprocal inhibition of mutually exclusive innervations ; it is now for consideration what origin is to be ascribed to analogous sensations in the case of the other variety of tone. The answer to this may, I think, be found in the indisputable fact that the free exercise of muscular activity is intrinsically pleasant. Freud even goes so far as to reckon the muscles, in this respect, among the erogenous zones whose stimulation gives rise to 'sexual' pleasure. (Compare almost any account of the Freudian theory of Infantile Sexuality—a better name for which would be Infantile Sensuousness.) This fact is not only adequately supported by common experience but also accords with what we should expect on general grounds. Biological processes have certainly operated—whatever their mechanisms—in such a way as to produce organisms so constituted physiologically that activities of survival value, or stimulations provocative of such activities, are pleasant and, in general, positively toned. In this category unimpeded muscular movement can certainly be reckoned. An infant who derived no satisfaction from the mere exercise of his limbs would never develop his muscles adequately, and his chances of survival would be correspondingly diminished. This seems competent to explain how the evocation of 'harmonious' systems of ideas is as productive of affective tone as is that of 'conflicting' systems.

Why one kind of somatic sensation should produce the state of mind we call pleasantly toned, while another produces the oppositely toned state is, and must remain, an insoluble problem ; but this equally applies to the question of why one kind of sensation should produce the state of mind we call ' seeing,' while another produces that very different state we call ' hearing.'

I feel that I may reasonably claim some measure of support for this somatic view of the origin of affective tone, from the fact that the latter seems inseparably bound up with physiological changes in a way which the purely cognitive and ' intellectual ' elements of mental activities are not. Whenever we study any somatic change, such as involuntary muscular movements, or respiration, or heart-beat, or secretions of glands, or the psycho-galvanic reflex simultaneously with changes in affective tone we find a correspondence between the two sets of phenomena, and it seems probable that if we could apply perfect quantitative methods to the study of this correspondence we should find a one-to-one correlation. But wherever there is a significant correlation between two series of phenomena it is necessary to suppose either that one is the cause of the other or that both are due to the operation of a common cause. The former is the simpler view and, in this case, supports the considerations I have brought forward above.

There are one or two minor points which harmonise with this view and which may conveniently be dealt with here. The first is the fact that the affective tone of a mental state is not amenable to direct introspection ; so soon as we try to attend to it, it vanishes and is gone. This would be a necessary consequence of its proceeding from relations between systems of ideas. For the effort to attend to the affective tone involves *ipso facto* a reorientation of the field of attention and, therefore, a disturbance of the relation responsible for the tone.

The second is that the affective intensity of the mental state corresponding to a reaction often appears to be determined by the ease with which that reaction can be carried out. Thus Dr Rivers says :

> " There seems to be little doubt that fear becomes especially pronounced when there is interference with, or even the prospect of interference with, the process of fleeing, and the possibility cannot be excluded that the normal and unimpeded flight of animals from danger is not accompanied by the emotion of fear." [1]

This is precisely what we should expect on the assumption that affective tone is the product of conflict or harmony between the different conative tendencies which are evoked by a given situation and which oppose or reinforce one another according to whether the motor reactions which they foreshadow and subliminally innervate are incompatible or not. In free and unimpeded flight devoid of even imagined obstruction—a state which is practically unobtainable I imagine—there is only one conative tendency, only one set of innervations going on ; no opposed and incompatible reaction is foreshadowed—consequently there is no conflict.

It is probable that the implications scattered throughout the preceding pages will have made clear the relation of the antithesis of ' pleasant '

[1] *Instinct and the Unconscious*, p. 57.

and ' unpleasant ' to that of ' positive ' and ' negative ' affective tone. I may, however, conveniently add a few words on the point. Pleasant and unpleasant is the original and fundamental distinction from which the other is genetically derived. The relation is precisely the same as that between Freud's ' pleasure-pain ' and ' reality ' principles. On this subject Ernest Jones writes :

" The former represents the primary, original form of mental activity and is characteristic of the earliest' stages of human development, both in the individual and in the race. . . . Its main attributes are a tendency, on the one hand, to avoid pain and disagreeableness of whatever kind, and, on the other, a never-ceasing demand for immediate gratification . . . it is, in other words, ruled entirely by the hedonic pleasure-pain (*Lust—Unlust*) principle. . . . The function of the latter (reality principle) is to adapt the organism to the exigencies of reality, to subordinate the imperious demand for immediate gratification, and to replace this by a more distant but more permanently satisfactory one. It is thus influenced by social, ethical and other external considerations that are ignored by the earlier principle." [1]

This is, of course, somewhat loosely expressed but it sufficiently shows the nature of the relation in question. At first, pleasant tone is synonymous with positive and unpleasant with negative ; but so soon as experience begins to

[1] *Papers on Psycho-analysis*, Second Edition, 1920, p. 3.

operate through association, the reactions and mental processes of the organism begin to be oriented not only by immediate but also by ultimate gratification. The two may, and frequently do, coincide, but when they do not— when ' unpleasant ' ideas are positively toned, it is because past experiences, conserved as memories and brought into play by association, give rise to greater conflict if the ideas in question are not present to consciousness than if they are.

One merit of this view of affective tone is the ease with which it can be brought into line with the mechanism of ' repression.' It seems fairly clear that the state of conflict produced by the reciprocal inhibition of mutually exclusive conative tendencies cannot persist indefinitely, for so long as it lasts the organism is immobilised, so to speak, and its activities suspended ; the condition is one of unstable equilibrium, very easily disturbed. But this disturbance means simply that of the two conflicting systems one is displaced from consciousness and succeeded by another. This I conceive to be the general process whereby the appearance and disappearance of ideas in consciousness is brought about. Of this process repression is but one aspect, although the word is commonly used in a much more limited sense and as if it referred to a distinct mechanism.

It will almost certainly be objected at this point that repressed ideas are by definition, ideas which are never present to consciousness at all. This is perfectly true in some cases, but it does not really invalidate my view. In the first place, the fact that repressed ideas are never brought to consciousness does not mean that they *never have been* present thereto and I cannot see my way to agreeing with those who maintain this, for I completely fail to understand how these authorities account for the presence of the ideas concerned in the mind at all.

But, granting that they have got there somehow, my view continues to hold good, for we know that although such ideas never come into the full focus of attention, so to speak, and never reach the centre of the field of consciousness, they do on occasion approach the ' marginal fringe.' (These metaphorical expressions are very unsatisfactory, but they seem to be unavoidable.) It is only by supposing this to be so that we can account for the fact that marked affective tone is produced whenever a situation contains elements which are associated with the repressed ideas. It is on this fact alone that the word-association test is founded ; if it were not so, we could never get on the track of ' complexes ' by observing the phenomena evoked by the stimulus-words.

A further analogy naturally suggests itself here. Repressed ' negatively ' toned ideas behave very much as electrically charged bodies would do in the presence of another similarly and intensely changed body. They are repelled by the latter, but so long as they are far removed from it the repulsion is negligible, while if for any external reason they are drawn towards it the repulsion rapidly increases. Somewhat similarly, repressed ideas, which would be productive of negative tone if present in the field of consciousness, are, so to speak, innocuous so long as they remain beyond the marginal fringe and lie buried in the unconscious. But so soon as external circumstances (*e.g.* the stimulus-words) arouse them and tend to draw them into consciousness, conflict is set up and negative tone results.

I regard repression, as commonly understood, as no more than a part of the general process whereby systems of ideas are displaced from consciousness, or fail fully to accede to it, as a result of the conflict between their conative elements and those forming part of other dominant systems. The questions of why those other systems are ' dominant ' is, of course, very important but it would take us too far to discuss it here.

I ought also to touch on the question of whether it is really legitimate to speak of affective tone as the *cause* of mental changes. Strictly speaking, I doubt whether it is ; the changes and the tone are alike produced by a common cause—conflict or harmony of the kind discussed above, to wit—and perhaps neither can properly be regarded as the cause of the other. In practice, of course, this distinction is insignificant, since there is—according to my view—a one-to-one correlation between the conflict or harmony and the affective tone. But, apart from this I am inclined to think that affective tone is, if anything, the more fundamental of the two, for the potential reactions which harmonise or conflict have their *raison d'être* in adaptation to environment for failure in which unpleasant tone is the immediate penalty and the immediate motive power for readjustment.

Finally, I wish to point out that although I believe the account of the origin of affective tone which I have given in this chapter to be on approximately the right lines, the correctness or otherwise of my theoretical views has no bearing at all on whatever value my experimental results may possess. The main concept of positive and negative tone is founded on purely empirical evidence and neither its existence nor its mode of operation is affected by any theories we may construct as to its origin.

It is a matter of experimental fact that *something* (which we may as well call ' affective tone,' but which could equally well be referred to by any other symbol) can be measured by means of the psycho-galvanic reflex and exerts an influence on the accession of ideas to consciousness. This influence may work in either of two opposite directions and its cause must therefore be of two opposite kinds. Positive and negative merely happen to be convenient symbols for referring to these two varieties of the cause. If, as psychologists, we wish to study the ways in which the content of consciousness varies, we can safely use these empirically observed facts and the symbols for referring to them without in any way committing ourselves to the acceptance of any particular theoretical doctrine as to the true nature or origin of the facts.

CHAPTER VIII

SUMMARY

I MAY conveniently conclude this book with a brief summary of its principal contents.

In the first chapter a brief account is given of my personal attitude towards the general theory of Emotion and Affective Tone. I propose to reserve the former term for reference to specific emotions, such as Fear or Rage, and to use the latter to denote the general emotional quality of mental states. Identifying myself in the main with the James-Lange theory of emotion and with Professor M'Dougall's view of the relation between this and Instinct, I deal briefly with one or two criticisms of the former and explain how this theory seems to me to fit in with Professor M'Dougall's views.

I conclude with a few remarks on the psychogalvanic reflex and the word-association test as such.

In Chapter II I describe experiments to determine the influence of Affective Tone on Memory. The psycho-galvanic reflex, the reaction time and the reproduction test are used to detect and measure affective tone elicited by word-association tests, and periodic reproduction of learned words gives a measure of their memory value. Co-ordination of the two sets of data shows that a marked influence is exerted by affective tone on memory, especially when the reflex is used. In this case the influence may be exerted in either of two opposite directions, whence the existence of two opposite kinds of tone is deduced. These are named positive and negative respectively. The indications of reaction time and reproduction test are also discussed.

In Chapter III I investigate the properties of complex-indicators and combinations thereof. Eight combinations are possible and I compute the mean memory value for each such combination. It is shown that the reproduction test is the best complex-indicator in the pathological sense and the properties of the various combinations (some of which indicate one kind of tone and others the opposite kind) are worked out both qualitatively and quantitatively. The results show a remarkable quantitative concordance.

In Chapter IV I apply the foregoing results to the study of the different verbal forms which the association may take. I adopt a system of classification slightly different from that of Jung and give theoretical and (subsequently) experimental justification for the alteration. It is found that different verbal forms have, on the average, widely different affective qualities and again there is found to be good agreement both between qualitative and quantitative results and between these and theoretical considerations. A ' check back ' on to memory values confirms the reliability of the methods used and the ' innerness ' of the association is surmised to be chiefly an index of negative tone.

In Chapter V I describe experiments to show that the association test in conjunction with the psycho-galvanic reflex may be used as a criterion of individuality. The coefficient of correlation between the reactions of any individual on different occasions is shown to be on the average much higher than that between the reactions of different individuals to the same—suitably chosen—list of stimulus-words. Possible applications of this method are suggested, notably with respect to the phenomena of hypnosis and multiple personality.

In Chapter VI I describe experiments on the effects of alcohol on the psycho-galvanic reflex and the word-association test. The first effect noted is the diminution of the absolute magnitude of the mean reflex. The variability of reactions is also diminished. Analysis of the reactions and verbal associations by the technique developed in Chapters III and IV shows that, under the influence of alcohol, there is a tendency to regress to a more primitive, all-or-none, or ' protopathic ' type of reaction.

In Chapter VII I return to the theoretical discussion of affective tone. I point out that any system of classification is permissible, provided it is useful for the purpose in hand, but the contention is put forward that the distinction between positive and negative tone as already defined is fundamental to the psychologist. An attempt is made to account for the origin of the two varieties of tone in terms of the nervous excitations accompanying the organic adjustments evoked in response to the contemporary situation.

APPENDIX I

REACTIONS OF A TYPICAL SUBJECT

No.	Stimulus Word.	Reaction Word.	R.T.	Galvanometer. From	To	Diff.	No.	Stimulus Word.	Reaction Word.	R.T.	Galvanometer. From	To	Diff.
1	Head	Hand	10	20	34	14	51	Frog	Whip [1]	10	60	66	6
2	Green	Sea	11	23	38	15	2	Try	Judge	12	58	61	3
3	Water	Cave	10	25	28	3	3	Hunger	Thirst	10	58	59	1
4	Sing	Song	9	22	32	10	4	White	Black	12	57	59	2
5	Dead	Alive	15	22	44	22	5	Child	Baby	14	56	77	21
6	Long	Short	8	30	34	4	6	Speak	Sing	11	64	64	0
7	Ship	Sail	9	27	30	3	7	Pencil	Write	11	61	62	1
8	Make	Blouse	10	25	33	8	8	Sad	Sorrow	18	60	63	3
9	Woman	Child	7	24	29	5	9	Plum	Apple	15	58	58	0
10	Friend	Girl	15	21	43	22	60	Marry	Wedding	20	55	72	17
1	Cook	Meat	20	31	36	5	1	Home	House	14	58	59	1
2	Ask	What?	10	28	33	5	2	Nasty	Bitter	20	56	68	12
3	Cold	Hot	8	30	44	14	3	Glass	Looking	12	61	62	1
4	Stalk	Flour	8	35	36	1	4	Fight	Dogs	10	56	65	9
5	Dance	Music	9	30	43	13	5	Wine	?	15	58	77	19
6	Village	Town	8	32	37	5	6	Big	Tree	12	64	66	2
7	Pond	Lake	7	31	34	3	7	Carrot	Turnip	10	63	64	1
8	Sick	Ill	9	30	54	24	8	Give	Present	10	72	80	8
9	Proud	Humble	10	42	53	11	9	Doctor	Ill	11	62	63	1
20	Bring	Carry	10	39	47	8	70	Travel	?	11	61	63	2
1	Ink	Letter	9	39	49	10	1	Flower	Iris	12	61	66	5
2	Angry	Fierce	8	38	48	10	2	Beat	Horse	15	60	68	8
3	Needle	Thread	9	37	40	3	3	Box	Journey	11	61	65	4
4	Swim	Sea	10	36	43	7	4	Old	Young	10	60	62	2
5	Go	When?	9	36	44	8	5	Family	Many	12	59	66	7
6	Blue	Red	14	36	49	13	6	Wait	Station	10	60	62	2
7	Lamp	Oil	12	38	42	4	7	Cow	Bull	10	59	60	1
8	Carry	Basket	18	37	41	4	8	Name	Letter	15	58	61	3
9	Bread	Butter	9	35	39	4	9	Luck	Cards	11	58	63	5
30	Rich	Poor	8	36	38	2	80	Horse	Ride	9	60	63	3
1	Tree	Leaf	9	36	37	1	1	Table	Dinner	9	59	60	1
2	Jump	Leap	8	34	41	7	2	Work	Hard	10	58	58	0
3	Pity	Sorrow	13	34	50	16	3	Brother	Sister	8	57	58	1
4	Yellow	Flower	16	40	47	7	4	Afraid	Fire	9	57	66	9
5	Street	?	12	40	47	7	5	Love	Children	7	60	101	41
6	Bury	Dead	10	41	46	5	6	Chair	Seat	11	85	85	0
7	Salt	Sugar	8	40	42	2	7	Worry	Why?	15	80	96	16
8	Dress	White	14	41	48	7	8	Kiss	Pleasant	8	81	109	28
9	Habit	Riding	10	40	43	3	9	Motor	Far	11	86	87	1
40	Pray	God	11	40	62	22	90	Clean	Polish	14	85	86	1
1	Money	Gold	8	52	55	3	1	Bag	Carry	10	83	85	2
2	Silly	Stupid	14	48	55	7	2	Choice	What?	15	82	88	6
3	Book	Poetry	11	47	50	3	3	Bed	Comfy	9	81	82	1
4	Despise	Contempt	12	46	51	5	4	State	England	10	79	82	3
5	Finger	Hand	10	46	49	3	5	Happy	Very	10	78	89	11
6	War	Sorrow	14	46	52	6	6	Shut	Door	10	77	77	0
7	Bird	Sing	9	47	49	2	7	Wound	Painful	11	78	84	6
8	Walk	Run	14	47	53	6	8	Evil	Doing	12	80	82	2
9	Paper	Parchment	11	48	54	6	9	Divorce	Court	17	77	86	9
50	Wicked	Man	14	54	72	18	100	Insult	Injury	12	77	82	5

[1] Misunderstood as "Flog."

APPENDIX II

A NOTE ON THE USE OF THE PSYCHO-GALVANIC REFLEX

ONE of the chief difficulties connected with the use of the psycho-galvanic reflex is that of making comparable with one another the reactions observed in different subjects and on different occasions. It might be supposed that the absolute magnitude of the reflex produced by such physical stimuli as pricks, burns, sudden noises and so forth, would afford an indication of the comparative 'emotivity' [1] of the subject concerned, and that this might be used as a 'vocational test' for occupations demanding self-control. But it was soon realised that factors other than emotivity greatly affect the absolute magnitude of the reflex which is, therefore, of small value as a test of that quality.

It is with this question of the comparability of reactions that the following observations are mainly concerned.

The phenomenon appears to be a very complex one and we are at present far from a thorough understanding of its mechanism. There seem to be, for instance, at least two clearly distinguishable forms of the reflex; first, a change in the effective resistance offered by the skin to the passage of an electric current and, second, a generated electro-motive force which is independent of any current applied *ab extra*.

---

[1] 'Emotivity' being here used to denote liability to react to an exciting stimulus.

APPENDIX

Of these two varieties the former is certainly a skin effect, though whether it is due to a change within the skin itself or to a change of polarisation at its surface is not yet clear. It is with this form that I shall concern myself below.

Many methods have been used for studying the reflex. Following Waller, I myself have always used a Wheatstone's bridge and D'Arsonval galvanometer in conjunction with two zinc-plate electrodes, covered with wash-leather and soaked in a concentrated solution of common salt ; these were applied to the palm and back of the subject's left hand which thus formed the external resistance of the bridge.

The following factors appear to be involved in determining the absolute magnitude of the galvanometer deflexion produced by a given stimulus :

(i) The intensity of the emotion actually evoked.
(ii) The proportion of it which finds expression through those efferent channels which innervate the skin-mechanisms responsible for the reflex.
(iii) The responsiveness of the skin to such innervation.[1]
(iv) The initial resistance of the skin.
(v) The sensitivity of the galvanometer.
(vi) The magnitude of the fixed resistances of the bridge.
(vii) The E.M.F. applied to the bridge.

Of these, (i) is the quantity which we wish to measure, (v), (vi) and (vii) are easily kept constant or, if not, suitable corrections can be made on their account. Of the remainder, (iv) can readily be measured, and I deal below with the appropriate correction for it, but (ii) and (iii) are variables for which, at present, no allowance can be made.

I propose to deal here with the question of what correction should be applied to compensate for variations in the initial resistance of the skin.

[1] I think it probable that this factor may, for all practical purposes, be subsumed under (ii) or (iv) or both.

This point is of importance for two reasons. First : even if we cannot eliminate all the causes of variation, other than (i) above, between different subjects, it is desirable to remove as many as we can, both with a view to closer study of those which remain and in order to reduce the amount of fortuitous variations to be neutralised by the use of such statistical methods as may be necessary. Second : if we are studying the behaviour of the same subject on different occasions we shall wish to make the results obtained as comparable as possible with respect to (i) and we may for the present assume that (ii), at least, and perhaps (iii) are not likely to vary greatly in the same subject from time to time.

One of the obvious results of a difference in resistance between two subjects will be that a heavier current will be passed through the subject of lower resistance than through the one of higher resistance (assuming the E.M.F. on the bridge to be kept constant).

It is easy to show experimentally that, in general, the greater the current passed through the subject, the greater is the absolute magnitude of his reactions. The question then arises whether this increased reaction is due simply to what I may call ' normal ' electrical causes or whether, as has been suggested by Prideaux, the heavier current produces some definite effect on the subject of such a nature as to increase his ' irritability ' quite apart from the increased deflexion which would be expected on purely electrical grounds. In other words, can the living subject be treated, so far as differences of initial skin resistance are concerned, as if he were an inanimate resistance whose changes we were observing ?

This would be easy to determine if we could apply standard stimuli to subjects of different resistances and measure the deflexions produced. This procedure, however, appears to me impracticable, partly because a stimulus of small emotional import to one subject may arouse intense emotion in another and partly on account of possible and unknown effects due to the factors (ii) and (iii).

These difficulties can, however, be largely surmounted by the use of appropriate statistical methods.

In connexion with the experiments on memory and affective tone described in Chapter II, I had occasion to apply a word-association test of 100 words to 50 different subjects, and to compute the mean resistance of each for the period of the test. I therefore first calculated the coefficient of correlation between the mean galvanometer deflexion and the mean resistance for these 50 subjects. Its value was $-\cdot497$; that is to say, there is a strong tendency, as we would expect, for deflexions to increase as resistance decreases.

On general grounds it seemed probable that initial resistance and the deflexion produced by a given stimulus would be connected by a relation of the form

$$R^x D = K$$

when R is the initial resistance, D the deflexion and K a constant. I therefore calculated the values of the coefficient of variation for the expression, $R^x D$, for this series of 50 subjects, giving x the values 0, 1 and 2 successively.

The resulting values are :

x	C of V,
0	$\cdot656$,
1	$\cdot572$,
2	$\cdot704$.

These values lie on the curve $V = \cdot098x^2 - \cdot182x + \cdot656$, which has a minimum at the point $x = \cdot925$; $V = \cdot5717$.

That is to say, the effect on the absolute magnitude of deflexions, of differing resistances of the subjects, can be *more perfectly removed by multiplying the deflexions by $R^{.925}$—which is substantially equal to R—than by any other power of R.*

(It may be noted that the improvement effected by using the expression $R^{.925}D$ instead of RD is inappreciable, for the coefficient of variation only changes from ·572 to ·5717.)

As a check on this, I substituted a resistance box for the subject and obtained by direct calibration the deflexions corresponding to a constant percentage decrease in resistances of 1, 2, 3, 4, 5, 6, 7, 8, 9 and 10 thousand ohms. Similar treatment of these gave an optimum value for x of approximately ·9. We may therefore conclude that so far as variations of initial skin resistance are concerned, the subject does behave in substantially the same way as an inanimate resistance, and that the differences observed as the effect of passing a larger or smaller current through the subject are wholly due to normal electrical causes and not to any further effect of the current upon the subject himself.

It is not always necessary to apply this correction ; but in cases where it is desirable to do so, the inconvenience of actually multiplying each deflexion by the resistance of the subject can be obviated by any one of the three methods described below.

(i) If we take a subject of resistance 1000 ohms, say, as ' standard ' and use for such a subject a galvanometer shunt of x ohms selected so as to give deflexions of suitable size for ordinary stimuli (producing a decrease of resistance of about 2·5–3·0%), it is easy to obtain by calculation or, preferably, by direct calibration, the values of the shunts which will give the same deflexion for the same percentage decrease of resistance in the case of subjects of resistances 2000, 3000, 4000, etc., ohms. These values can be plotted graphically as ordinates against resistances as abscissæ

APPENDIX

and the shunt appropriate to a subject of any resistance can be read off from the resulting graph.

(ii) Another method is to use no shunt on the galvanometer but to control the magnitude of the deflexions by varying the E.M.F. applied to the bridge by means of a potentiometer. Here, again, the best procedure will be to calibrate the apparatus directly by substituting a resistance box for the subject, balancing resistances of 1, 2, 3, 4, 5, etc., thousand ohms on the bridge, reducing each of these when balanced by the same percentage—2·5 say—and adjusting the potentiometer so as to give the same deflexion in each case. Potentiometer adjustments can then be plotted against resistances as before.

(iii) A third method, which has the advantage that it requires considerably less apparatus than either of the foregoing, is to abolish the use of the bridge altogether and to employ a modification of Binswanger's arrangement described in Jung's *Studies in Word Association*, p. 446. The subject, battery and electrodes are here placed in series and no bridge is used.[1]

When the subject is at rest and not stimulated, there will, of course, be an initial steady deflexion of the galvanometer. Assuming that the resistance of the latter and of the remainder of the circuit is small compared with that of the subject, and that the galvanometer deflexions are proportional to the current over the range in question, the deflexion will increase by a percentage equal to that by which the subject's resistance decreases

Thus, for a subject of resistance 5000 ohms, the initial deflexion will be twice as great as for one of 10,000 ohms, and so will the added deflexion corresponding to any given stimulus.

[1] An alternative arrangement combining the advantages of this with those of the bridge mentioned has been described by Prideaux (*Brain*, 1920, XLIII, 50-73).

THE MEASUREMENT OF EMOTION

If we interpose a potentiometer between the battery and the circuit, we can always pass the same current through the subject, thereby producing a constant initial deflexion and constant subsequent deflexions for the same percentage decrements in the subject's resistance, whatever the absolute magnitude of the latter may be. This is what is required.

The only disadvantage of this method is that the galvanometer always starts with a large deflexion of which only a small percentage increase is observed as the result of stimuli. In its simpler form it has, however, been successfully used by Binswanger, Veraguth and others, and its simplicity and cheapness are very much in its favour.

As I have observed above, it is not always necessary to apply a correction for the resistance of the subject by any of these means or by direct multiplication. The way in which results are handled and the form in which they are expressed should depend upon the objects of the experiments. Thus, if we are using the reflex merely as a 'complex indicator' in a word-association test—as a preliminary to psycho-analytic treatment, for example—no corrections of any sort need be applied, for all that concerns us is the *relative* degree of emotion evoked by the various stimulus words. If, on the other hand, we are seeking to ascertain which words of a list, or which members of a series of other stimuli provoke most emotion, on the average, in a given class of subjects, it will be best to express the reaction to each stimulus as a percentage of the mean reaction of the subject concerned for all the stimuli. Thus, if ten stimuli are applied to a given subject with the following results :

Stimulus	A	B	C	D	E	F	G	H	I	K
Reaction	7	3	9	14	2	11	8	6	12	5

of which reactions the arithmetic mean is 7·7, we

should express the results for every such subject as follows :

Stimulus	A	B	C	D	E	F	G	H	I	K
Reaction	91	39	117	182	26	143	104	78	156	65

(% of mean)

This eliminates not only variations due to resistance but also the danger of the results being unduly influenced by excessively large or small reactions, of whatever origin, on the part of a single subject.

Whether the arithmetic or the probable mean should be used will depend on circumstances ; in nearly all cases the latter is preferable. But if we wish to compare the behaviour of different classes of subjects with respect to the psycho-galvanic reflex in general, it will be necessary to apply the correction for resistance. For the classes may differ by virtue of the factors (ii) and (iii) mentioned on p. 171 above, and this may be important. For instance, if we are comparing normal with mentally deficient persons, it may be, as is suggested by some as yet unpublished experiments by Prideaux, that the latter persons give very small reactions to all classes of stimuli because only a small proportion of the emotion aroused finds expression through the mechanisms responsible for the reflex, or because they have skins of resistance much higher than the normal, or because they really feel less—*i.e.* less emotion is actually aroused.

If the uncorrected results were simply averaged for a number of such defective persons and compared with the similarly treated results for normal persons, we could form no definite conclusions on the subject. Whereas, if due allowance is made for variations in skin resistance, any difference between the size of the reactions given by the two classes of subject can either be ascribed to this cause or, when it is eliminated, shown to be due to one or more of the others.

M

Finally, inasmuch as the phenomenon consists essentially in a lowering of the resistance of the skin, and as the percentage decrease of resistance appears to be, very approximately, directly proportional to the intensity of the emotion aroused, it is desirable that all results which are published with a view to comparison with those obtained by other experimenters should be expressed in terms of percentage decrement of resistance or, at least, that sufficient data should be given to enable the results to be reduced to these terms. Absolute deflexions are valueless for comparative purposes, as they depend so largely on the particular arrangement of apparatus used.

It may be of interest to note that in the case of the 50 subjects mentioned above the mean resistance for all subjects was 4400 ohms and the mean deflexion 7·32 mm. This corresponds, with my apparatus, to a decrement of resistance of about 2·3%.

APPENDIX III

A NOTE ON PROBABILITY

On pages 40 and 96 I have stated that the chance of the difference of two experimentally determined mean values being accidental had a certain approximate value.

I am indebted to my friend, Mr W. Hope-Jones of Eton College, for the following method of computing this chance:

"Given two means, x_1 (Probable Error $= \pm y_1$) and x_2 (Probable Error $= \pm y_2$), it is required to determine the probability that these two means differ as the result of chance and not by virtue of differing causation of origin.

"Write $y_1 = \cdot6745\, C_1$ and $y_2 = \cdot6745\, C_2$ so as to work in Standard Deviations instead of probable errors.

"Let $p = \dfrac{x_2 - x_1}{\sqrt{C_1^2 + C_2^2}}$ (x_2 being assumed greater than x_1).

Then the chance that the mean which has proved to be the greater is really less than the other is

$$\frac{\displaystyle\int_{p}^{\infty} C^{-\frac{x^2}{2}}\, dx}{\displaystyle\int_{-\infty}^{\infty} C^{-\frac{x^2}{2}}\, dx}.$$

"A table of the values of this function is given in Yule's *Statistics* and the actual values of the chances given in Chapters II and IV have been computed therefrom."

179

APPENDIX IV

PSYCHO-PHYSICAL QUANTA

IN the course of a minor investigation which led to nothing worth recording, I had occasion to work out a frequency curve for the magnitudes of the psycho-galvanic reflexes given by my twenty-seven most reliable subjects. In order to get over the difficulty of the absolute magnitudes of the deflexions given by different subjects not being comparable, I expressed each deflexion as a percentage of the mean deflexion given by the individual concerned and classified the resulting data in percentage groups. That is to say, I counted in each case the number of reactions which fell between 0% and 10% of the mean, between 10% and 20% and so on. The results were :

Percentage Class.[1]	Frequency.	Percentage Class.	Frequency.
0-10	168	130-140	104
10-20	66	140-150	87
20-30	162	150-160	55
30-40	91	160-170	53
40-50	151	170-180	40
50-60	153	180-190	55
60-70	182	190-200	35
70-80	123	200-210	29
80-90	204	210-220	24
90-100	144	220-230	30
100-110	165	230-240	18
110-120	141	240-250	17
120-130	100	250-260	17
		Over 260%	99
		Total . . .	2513

[1] For the sake of convenience I shall henceforward refer to class 0%-10% as 'class 0,' to class 10%-20% as 'class 10' and so forth.

APPENDIX

The frequencies above class 250-260 were too small to be of interest.

These figures are very remarkable. I do not propose to describe their full analysis in detail here for their most striking characteristics can be verified by inspection.

The first point to be noted is that they are clearly periodic. The frequencies in the different classes are, in general, alternately high and low; that is to say, they oscillate with a 20% period.

Secondly, there are exceptions to this rule. The most notable of these is class 50, but there is another breakdown in the neighbourhood of class 120. If the actual magnitudes of the oscillations be analysed with due regard to the fact that they must be regarded as superimposed on a smooth frequency distribution curve of approximately normal type, this alternate increase and decrease of the oscillations becomes very apparent. In my opinion the chance of this second periodicity being accidental is very remote and an approximate calculation indicates that it is not larger than 1 in 1200. The curve corresponding to these values is, therefore, a periodic curve compounded of at least two periodic components.

Thirdly, it should be noted that after the oscillations die away (e.g. in the neighbourhood of class 50) they reappear in the same phase. This is important because it disposes of the possibility that the effect is due to grouping in 10% classes material which is really distributed periodically in classes of some other size. If, for example, the reactions really tended to concentrate about the values 0%, 25%, 50%, 75%, etc., of their means the oscillations would behave substantially as they actually do up to and including class 50, but thereafter classes 70, 90, etc., would be large and classes 60, 80 and 100 would be small.

Consequently the frequencies seem to represent

a compound periodic curve formed by the combination of two independent periodic causes which produce an effect reminiscent of the 'beats' generated by two sinusoidal wave-motions of different frequencies.

It is this double periodicity which is alone worthy of comment, for simple oscillations could easily be accounted for by the nature of the material itself. If, for example, a subject gave reactions consisting exclusively of the magnitudes 0, 1, 2, 3, 4, 5, 6, 7, 8, 9 and 10 and if his mean reaction were very nearly 5 (between 4·9 and 5·1 say), it is obvious that the frequency distribution curve would show a 20% periodicity, for all reactions would be 0, 20, 40, 60, 80, 100, 120, 140, 160, 180 or 200% of the mean. Now it so happens that the material available in this connexion consisted largely of small integers and that several of the means were in the neighbourhood of 5, and it is therefore not improbable that the 20% periodicity might be due to this cause. I have tried to check this by determining whether, with the actual means in question, a random collection of small integers would tend to concentrate at 20% intervals, and there is no doubt that there is at least a slight tendency to do so. We may therefore ascribe one of the periodic components to the nature of the material.

On the other hand, I do not see how we are to account for the second periodic component on these lines. In order to do so we should have to suppose that the means were themselves grouped closely around two values and that both sets tended to produce periodic frequency distribution curves of different periods. Of this I can find no evidence at all, and I therefore find it necessary to look in some other direction for the cause of the second periodic component.

The only promising hypothesis seems to me to be to suppose that the relation between intensity of stimulus and magnitude of response is not smooth and continuous but is of a 'quantal' nature. I suggest, that is to say, that the energy responsible for the reaction is not liberated continuously to an extent proportional throughout to the strength of the stimulus but in instalments or 'quanta.'

Thus stimuli below a certain value would liberate no energy and the reaction would be *nil*. When this value is surpassed, energy to the value of 1 unit (or, more strictly, n units) is liberated, but no more than this is set free whatever the intensity of the stimulus unless it surpasses another 'landmark' of intensity when 2 units (or $2n$ units) are liberated, and so on. If this indication of the existence of psycho-physical 'quanta' be true, it seems to me likely to prove of great importance to physiological psychology and to psycho-physics.

And in spite of the fact that, so far as I am aware, the existence of psycho-physical quanta has never been either suspected or demonstrated before, the suggestion that the nervous system works in this way need not, I think, occasion much surprise.

It has long been realised that, like the rest of the body, it is discontinuous (cellular) in its essential structure. The unit is the 'neurone,' and it is a common practice to speak of the potential energy of a neurone being converted into kinetic energy by the incidence of a stimulus from some source or other. If the views implied by such phrases are correct it is clear that the conception of quanta of nervous energy is an almost necessary corollary. Again, if we consider the structure of synaptic junctions and of neurones possessing multiple processes which approximate to a multiplicity of other neurones, it seems almost inevitable to suppose that the conduction of nervous energy across such junctions or its 'irradiation' from such a neurone to its neighbours must proceed in a discontinuous fashion. In the first case the path of least resistance will first be used, then, if this is insufficient to cope with the energy potential, other paths of higher resistance will be found, each coming in more or less suddenly just as electricity 'sparks' suddenly across a gap between conductors when the electrical potential is sufficient. In the second case an analogous process may be supposed to operate, only here a number of different neurones will receive the discharge.

Something of this kind has already been observed to occur. Thus Sherrington has found that when in response to increased intensity of stimulus the flexion-reflex spreads from the knee to the hip, *the spread is not gradual but the hip flexion suddenly comes in.*[1] I am also told that indications of a quantal action have recently been obtained in the course of work on muscle and nerve.

I need hardly point out, I hope, that I fully realise the inconclusive nature of the evidence I have submitted   Unfortunately external circumstances prevent me from undertaking a fresh series of experiments in order definitely to settle the point at issue. I have therefore published these notes in the form of an Appendix in the hope that the phenomena noted may appear sufficiently interesting and suggestive to other workers to induce them to undertake an *ad hoc* investigation.

---

[1] *The Integrative Action of the Nervous System*, p. 76.   My italics.